ACUPUNCTURE

ff

ACUPUNCTURE
The modern scientific approach

Anthony Campbell MRCP(UK), FF Hom
Consultant Physican, Royal London Homoeopathic Hospital

faber and faber
LONDON · BOSTON

First published in 1987
by Faber and Faber Limited
3 Queen Square London WC1N 3AU

Filmset by Wilmaset, Birkenhead, Wirral
Printed in Great Britain by
Redwood Burn Ltd, Trowbridge, Wiltshire
All rights reserved

British Library Cataloguing in Publication Data

Campbell, Anthony
    Acupuncture: the modern scientific approach.
    1. Acupuncture
    I. Title
    615.8'92   RM184

ISBN 0–571–14652–X

CONTENTS

PREFACE

The word acupuncture means simply 'piercing with a sharp instrument' and so, by definition, refers to the use of needles to alleviate symptoms or cure disease. In most people's minds, however, it denotes the elaborate system of needle treatment that grew up in China over many hundreds of years, and it may come as a surprise to find that there is also a form of acupuncture that makes use of modern scientific concepts. This book is about modern 'scientific' acupuncture as opposed to the traditional system, but it would be a mistake to try to separate the two approaches too completely.

Western enthusiasts for traditional acupuncture often cling tenaciously to the ancient theories and practices, and make a point of emphasising how different acupuncture is from orthodox Western medicine. And, as happens with other forms of alternative medicine, acupuncture often becomes for such enthusiasts more than a mere method of treatment; it takes on a mystical aura, even though this was not a feature of the traditional system.

The ancient Chinese were remarkably pragmatic thinkers, and their modern descendants are certainly very receptive to new ideas in acupuncture; they have indeed introduced a number of innovations of their own. Certainly they are in no way hostile to studying acupuncture scientifically or to trying to explain it in modern physiological terms. They show, in fact, a notable degree of flexibility in their thinking, which is often not matched by Western advocates of traditional Chinese medicine.

In writing of 'scientific' acupuncture I do not mean to imply that we now have a full scientific understanding of the subject, but I do believe that it must in principle be possible to account for acupuncture physiologically. However, we certainly cannot do this yet, and by the time we can we shall undoubtedly have learnt a great deal about the way the nervous system works.

The main differences between the traditional and scientific versions of acupuncture are summarised in the following table.

Traditional	*Scientific*
Follows rules laid down in the past	Largely ignores the old rules
Is based on pre-scientific ideas	Is based on modern concepts of anatomy and physiology
Not mystical but appeals to Westerners interested in mysticism	No element of mysticism

The idea for this book grew out of the acupuncture courses for doctors that I have taught for a number of years at the Royal London Homoeopathic Hospital. When I first started to teach I looked for a suitable textbook, but I quickly realised that there was nothing that fully met my requirements. Most of the available books were on the traditional system, and the others were mostly 'cook books' – that is, lists of 'acupuncture points' to try in various disorders. I wanted to get away from both these approaches and instead to present students with what I thought, rightly or wrongly, were the essentials of the modern scientific approach. Since I could not find what I wanted I wrote my own notes, and the present book is in essence an expanded version of these.

The book is thus intended primarily for doctors and other health professionals interested in acupuncture, but I hope it will also be useful for non-medical readers who want to understand what acupuncture is and what it can offer. This is important, because it is an advantage if acupuncture patients do have some understanding of the treatment they are receiving. Probably for reasons to do with the way in which the nervous system is built, it seems to be necessary for patients at least to be willing to be treated by acupuncture and not to be too afraid of it if it is to succeed (although they do not need to *believe* in it; scepticism is not a problem, only fear or reluctance). In many branches of medicine it is not practical to try to write a book suitable for both doctors and lay people, but acupuncture differs from most of medicine in being essentially simple and therefore, in principle, accessible to people without a medical background. Even so, some use of medical terms is inevitable. This is specially true of Chapters 7 and 8, which deal with the practical aspects of treatment, and which are primarily intended for professionals.

Just because acupuncture is so practical, there are inevitable limitations attached to the attempt to write an acupuncture textbook. Acupuncture cannot be learnt from a book, any more than piano playing or cooking. Personal instruction is essential for all these skills. However, a book has its uses. No one can take in or remember all, or even most, of what is said in a lecture; even the most attentive student needs a text to which he can refer later. Besides, a book provides the opportunity to develop and expand certain ideas that can only be touched on briefly in lectures.

I should like to emphasise at the outset that this is simply one approach to scientific acupuncture. There is no single right way to practise acupuncture; every experienced medical acupuncturist has his or her own ideas and there is simply not enough firm knowledge available at present to allow confident statements about what should or should not be done. I claim only that the treatments I describe work in a substantial proportion of cases, but other doctors use different methods and these work too. It will be many years before it is possible to say which are the best procedures to use in specific circumstances.

To avoid offending the susceptibilities of female readers I should explain my use of pronouns. I have throughout usually referred to the doctor as 'he' and the patient as 'she', partly because this is in fact the situation most commonly encountered but chiefly because it saves considerable confusion.

ACKNOWLEDGEMENTS

I should like to thank Dr Felix Mann for giving me my first introduction to acupuncture. I also thank Dr Richard Petty for kindly supplying a number of valuable references. I am grateful to many colleagues for helpful discussions; to my students from whom I have learned much; and finally to the best instructors of all, my patients.

I thank Mrs Audrey Besterman for producing the line drawings in the book. Figure 9/1 was taken by Denis Nutley LRPS and both Figures, 9/1 and 9/2, were supplied by P. H. Medical, Weybridge, Surrey; I thank them all.

ADDENDUM: ACUPUNCTURE AND AIDS

There have so far been no reported cases of AIDS being transmitted by acupuncture needles. Nevertheless, public alarm about AIDS is now so great that the practice of re-using acupuncture needles is already diminishing rapidly among doctors and will probably soon be completely abandoned. The currently available disposable pre-sterilised needles are mostly of rather poor quality, but better ones (at increased cost) will doubtless come on the market soon.

In present circumstances, the only responsible advice that can be given is that acupuncture needles should be disposed of after use.

Chapter One
TRADITIONAL CHINESE MEDICINE

Crude forms of acupuncture seem to have been practised at various times in many parts of the world, but only in China did the technique attain the status of a major form of therapy, with a rich literature and elaborate theoretical basis. Even in China, however, acupuncture was never the only or even the main form of treatment; many more of the classical texts deal with herbalism than with acupuncture. To understand acupuncture one has to set it within the context of traditional Chinese medicine as a whole, and indeed it has to be seen against the background of Chinese science and philosophy in general.

The essential source book for ancient Chinese medical theory is the *Inner Classic of the Yellow Emperor* – the *Nei Ching*. This is a collection of texts by unknown authors compiled between 300 and 100 BC. Later writers commented on the *Nei Ching* to bring out and clarify its ideas or sometimes to add new ones. Without such commentaries the *Nei Ching* would be almost incomprehensible to modern readers. Modern textbooks are based on works written in the Ching (Manchu) period (1644–1911) and before that the Han period (202 BC to AD 220).

Chinese medical theory thus has a very long history and naturally many changes and developments occurred. Certain basic ideas, however, are constant and the most important of these is yin-yang polarity.

YIN AND YANG

The terms yin and yang are impossible to translate. Originally *yang* meant the sunny side of a slope or the north bank of a river, while *yin* meant the shady side of a slope or the south bank of a river. These meanings were later extended to cover a vast range of polarities, so that yang, for example, came to refer to heat, movement, vigour, increase, and upward or outward movement, while yin referred to cold, rest, passivity, decrease, and interior and downward movement. On the human level, yang is male, yin female.

It is essential to realise that although yin and yang are polar opposites they are not mutually exclusive. On the contrary, yang always contains at least a trace of yin and vice versa. This is indicated in the traditional yin-yang symbol by the fact that yang contains a small spot of yin and yin a small spot of yang (Fig. 1/1).

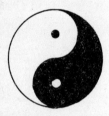

Fig. 1/1 Yin-yang symbol

This is a fascinating philosophical idea that carries many resonances. For example, in psychology it relates to the Jungian notion that none of us is wholly masculine or feminine but all contain something of both in our make-up. In physics, similarly, it can be applied to magnetism: if you cut a bar magnet in half you always produce both a north and a south magnetic pole, never a single north or south pole alone.

Yin and yang are not thought of as static entities but rather as dynamic forces that constantly interact with each other and transform themselves into each other. In the whole of nature, as well as in ourselves, there is an ever-changing flow of yang into yin and yin into yang.

Our state of health is thought to depend on the balance between yin and yang. If either preponderates more than it should the result may be disease, which is thus thought of as resulting from a dynamic imbalance. Treatment, similarly, is conceived of as a means of restoring the balance; the whole of classical acupuncture is concerned with this.

In addition to ideas derived from yin-yang polarity, the ancient Chinese physicians made use of a large number of anatomical and physiological concepts, including of course the famous 'points' and 'meridians', also certain substances such as *chi*.

Since these are important for an understanding of the traditional system of acupuncture we need to look at them in a little more detail.

SOME BASIC MEDICAL CONCEPTS

1. Chi

Chi is another untranslatable term. It is sometimes rendered as energy, but Chinese thought does not distinguish between matter and energy. It could perhaps be thought of as lying at the border between matter and energy, but it is impossible to define the concept clearly, partly because traditional Chinese thought does not seem to deal much in definitions. Chi is described dynamically, in terms of what it does. It sustains all kinds of movement and change, it protects against harmful influences, it transforms food into other substances as well as into chi itself, it holds organs in place and prevents excessive fluid loss, and it warms the body. It flows in special channels (the meridians) in conjunction with the blood; chi is yang, blood yin. The channels for chi and the blood vessels form one system. A fascinating feature of this scheme is that chi and blood were thought of as circulating in a pumped system; thus the ancient Chinese anticipated William Harvey's discovery of the circulation of the blood by hundreds of years (indeed, as early as the second century BC).

2. The organs

Chinese medicine recognises a number of internal organs, but though their names mostly correspond to organs described by Western anatomists their supposed functions are quite different. There are five yin organs (heart, lungs, spleen, liver and kidneys; the pericardium is sometimes included as well). There are six yang organs (gall bladder, stomach, small intestine, large intestine, urinary bladder and triple warmer).

3. Channels (meridians) and points (Fig. 1/2)

The term *meridian*, though widely used, is misleading; 'channels' is a better translation of the Chinese word (*ching*) since the idea is that there are subtle vessels running through the body to connect the various organs and to carry chi. Diagrams of the channels represent them as if they were lying on the surface of the body, but in fact they should be thought of as running at a variable depth inside the body and only coming to the surface at certain places. They have been compared to the Underground District Line, which at times runs below ground and at others emerges on the surface.

The acupuncture points mostly lie on the channels at places where they run near the surface, but a few points (the so-called extra-meridian points) are not situated on channels.

A total of 59 channels is described but of these only 14 possess acupuncture points. Of the 14, 12 are paired and 2 are midline, therefore unpaired.

Some 365 acupuncture points are described (the exact number varies slightly from source to source). In practice a much smaller number is used. The points all have names, which often sound poetic (Sea of Blood, Gate of Dumbness, Crooked Spring); these reflect their supposed functions. Western books on traditional acupuncture, however, use a more or less standardised numbering system instead of individual names.

The channels that possess acupuncture points are listed in the following table (see p. 8), with their commonly used Western abbreviations:

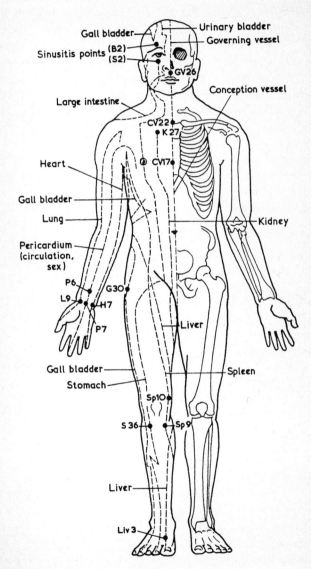

Fig. 1/2 The course of the main channels – front view

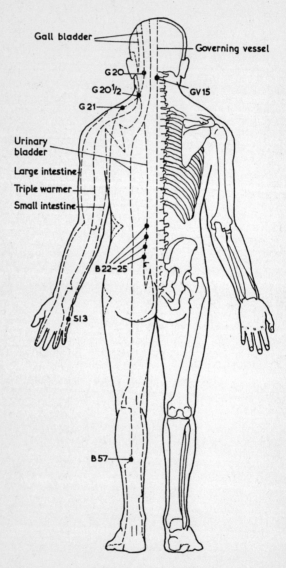

Gall bladder

Governing vessel

G 20

G 20½

GV 15

G 21

Urinary bladder

Large intestine

Triple warmer

Small intestine

B 22–25

SI 3

B 57

Fig. 1/2 The course of the main channels – back view

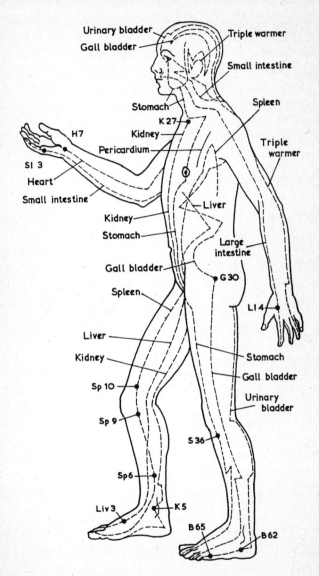

Fig. 1/2 The course of the main channels – lateral view

Paired
1. Lung (L)
2. Large Intestine (LI)
3. Stomach (S)
4. Spleen (Sp)
5. Heart (H)
6. Small Intestine (SI)
7. Urinary Bladder (B)
8. Kidney (K)
9. Pericardium (P) – also called Sex and Circulation
10. Triple Warmer (T)
11. Liver (Liv)
12. Gall Bladder (G)
Unpaired
13. Conception Vessel (CV)
14. Governing Vessel (GV)

The sequence used in the above table is that found in most books on traditional Chinese medicine because it corresponds to the way in which chi is supposed to flow. In order to grasp the overall picture, however, readers trained in Western anatomy will find it easier to adopt a different approach. If we ignore the traditional theory and instead regard the channels as if they were real anatomical structures that might be described in a modern textbook, we find that they can be arranged in two main classes: an *upper limb* group and a *lower limb* group. The upper limb group can be further subdivided into an anterior and a posterior subgroup, but this is more difficult in the lower limb.

The following table sets out this arrangement and also indicates the main areas in which the various channels run, together with the sequence of point numbering, distal-proximal or vice versa.

Certain features of this table should be particularly noted.
1. Some of the lower limb channels (G, S, and B) have a very long course and wide distribution, extending over the whole length of the body.
2. Certain channels cross each other, especially Liv and Sp.

3. G is the only truly lateral channel and B the only truly posterior channel.
4. For much of its course on the back B is doubled.

Channel	Situation	Distribution	Point Sequence
A. UPPER LIMBS			
Anterior group			
L	radial	shoulder/hand	prox-dist
P	median	shoulder/hand	prox-dist
H	ulnar	axilla/hand	prox-dist
Posterior group			
LI	radial	hand/face	dist-prox
T	median	hand/face	dist-prox
SI	ulnar	hand/face	dist-prox
B. LOWER LIMBS			
G	lateral	head/foot	prox-dist
S	anterior	head/foot	prox-dist
B	posterior	head/foot	prox-dist
K	post/med	foot/chest	dist-prox
Liv	medial	foot/chest	dist-prox
Sp	medial	foot/chest	dist-prox
C. MIDLINE			
CV	anterior	perineum/chin	inf-sup
GV	posterior	coccyx/upper lip	inf-sup

The five element theory

The yin-yang theory is the main foundation of Chinese medical theory. There is another theory which, though of lesser importance, receives a good deal of attention in Western books on traditional acupuncture. This is the so-called law of five elements. In fact, 'phases' would be a better rendering of the Chinese word than 'elements' because, as usual in Chinese thought, the concept is one of change and flow rather than of static substances. The five phases are Wood, Fire, Earth, Metal and Water, and these are related to the various organs and to one another in a complicated manner; the various inter-relationships are used to explain symptoms and decide how to treat them (Fig. 1/3).

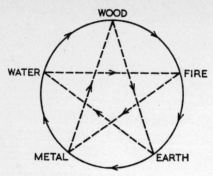

Fig. 1/3 Five element diagram

There is an apparent resemblance here to the Aristotelian-Galenic scheme of four elements (earth, air, fire and water) that was so influential in mediaeval European medicine, but there are important differences in the ways in which the two theories were regarded.

Modern Chinese books on acupuncture do not usually say much about the five element theory, perhaps because it is considered too abstruse; but it receives a good deal of attention in Western books on traditional acupuncture, perhaps because its very abstruseness makes it appear impressive and provides plenty of material for exposition.

5. Concepts of disease

Disease is held to be caused by three kinds of influence: environment, emotions and way of life. Way of life includes diet, physical activity and sexual activity; the principal environmental influences are wind, cold, heat and dampness. This is a truly holistic theory, but there is no real correspondence between these concepts and those of modern Western medicine, which is one reason why it is difficult to move between the two systems. A Western trained doctor, for example, would not know what to make of the statement that a patient was suffering from Internal Cold and required his kidney chi to be strengthened; equally, a traditional Chinese physician would not understand a diagnosis of chronic nephritis.

6. Methods of diagnosis

Like his Western counterpart, the traditional Chinese physician takes his patient's history and notes her general appearance and demeanour. Particular attention is paid to the tongue: its colour, coating, and so on, are recorded. The single most important examination, however, is that of the pulse. This is felt at the wrist, in three positions on each side and both superficially and deeply; this gives a total of twelve pulses, which are related to the twelve internal organs. (Some sources give even larger numbers of pulses.) A skilful physician is said to be able to derive an astonishing amount of information from the pulse alone, but learning the art requires thorough training, long experience, and the gift of intuition or sensitivity. Perhaps for this reason the art of pulse taking seems to receive comparatively little attention in modern Chinese schools of traditional medicine.

TREATMENT ACCORDING TO THE TRADITIONAL SYSTEM

A physician who follows the traditional system will take a history and carry out an examination in the manner I have outlined. He will then come to a decision about how to apply treatment. If this is to be acupuncture instead of (or as well as) a herbal prescription he will decide, mainly from the pulse, which organs require 'tonifying' or 'sedating', as the case may be. (The *five element theory* would be relevant here.)

In traditional acupuncture it was held to be essential to locate the acupuncture points with great precision. Indeed, in ancient times students were tested by confronting them with a bronze manikin in which the acupuncture points had been drilled. The manikin was coated with wax and then filled with water. The student, having listed the acupuncture points he would use to treat a given condition, would then be asked to insert needles in the appropriate places. If he was rewarded by a jet of water, well and good; otherwise he had failed.

Traditional Chinese physicians use a quite sophisticated method for describing the location of the acupuncture points. Because individuals vary in their bodily dimensions, the Chinese try to compensate for this by using a 'Chinese inch' or *chun*. There are various ways of measuring this but a common one is derived from the length of the middle joint in the patient's middle finger; acupuncture points can then be described as lying so many 'inches' from a particular landmark. The depth of the point is also specified in 'inches'. This is a good method in principle, although in practice it does not always lead to such precise location as might be hoped. Modern Chinese textbooks tend to follow the example set by Western writers on the subject and to superimpose the points on drawings of the skeleton.

The aim of the traditional treatment is to correct imbalances in the flow of chi. The underlying concept is essentially a hydraulic one, and the acupuncturist is something like an engineer, turning valves on and off to adjust the volume of the current and distribute it according to need. The traditional physician pays attention not only to the location of the acupuncture points but also to the manner of needling them. Great importance is attached to the concepts of 'tonification' and 'sedation'; certain points are held to be points that tonify or sedate, and there are also various different needling techniques that are used to produce these effects.

Having applied his treatment, the physician rechecks the pulses to see whether he has succeeded in balancing them. If not, he gives further treatment.

A great deal of attention is paid to obtaining various types of sensation from the patient, and the physician also experiences certain things as he manipulates the needle. These phenomena are supposed to be produced by tapping into the flow of chi and are said to be essential for successful treatment. Four typical sensations are described, and have been translated as numbness, fullness, heaviness and 'sourness' (a kind of muscular ache like that caused by over-exertion). These may be felt both locally and at some distance from the site of needling.

Traditional acupuncture is clearly a painstaking and time-consuming procedure and it is perhaps hardly surprising that in modern Chinese hospitals, with their enormous numbers of patients, the full system does not seem to be used very often.

Instead, the patients are treated collectively in large groups, purely on the basis of their symptoms or of a conventional medical diagnosis, without the benefit of a pulse diagnosis or the other traditional procedures. As a rule large numbers of needles are inserted, and electrical stimulation may be used.

The time at which treatment was applied was considered to be important in the traditional system. Indeed, the Chinese remarkably anticipated another modern discovery here: circadian rhythms. It is known today that a number of physiological functions follow a diurnal rhythm, waxing and waning throughout the 24 hours. Diseases, too, may follow a rhythmic course, sometimes within a 24-hour period, sometimes in longer cycles. Observations of this kind are to be found in the *Nei Ching*.

MOXIBUSTION

Moxibustion is a technique of treatment allied to acupuncture, in which moxa, a substance prepared from the leaves of plants of the *Artemisia* species, is burned to provide local heating. Moxibustion is generally held to be better for chronic disease, acupuncture for acute disease.

The moxa, which may be as small as a millet seed or as large as a cigar, is used in various ways. It may be held close to the skin, so that it warms it without burning it, or it may be placed on a layer of soya bean sauce, a slice of garlic, or a slice of ginger, to provide a measure of insulation. In some cases, however, a skin burn is deliberately inflicted, though this is said not to be too unpleasantly painful. The points at which moxa is applied are mostly the same as acupuncture points, but some are different.

TRADITIONAL ACUPUNCTURE IN THE LIGHT OF MODERN KNOWLEDGE

Traditional acupuncture is an enormously rich system of ideas that has existed for hundreds, even thousands, of years, and has served well for one of the subtlest and most intellectually sophisticated civilisations the world has seen. As we have it today, however, it is essentially a mediaeval system and from a modern scientific standpoint it is natural to ask whether it is objectively valid. In other words, do the channels, points, and so forth, really exist or not?

In 1963 a Korean anatomist, Kim Bonghan, published accounts of microscopical studies that showed certain corpuscles and thin ducts associated with them. These, he claimed, were the elusive acupuncture channels. Researchers in other countries who tried to repeat this work, however, were unsuccessful, and there seems to be no real doubt that Kim Bonghan was mistaken (see Needham and Gwei-Djen, 1980).

It is often said that the reality of acupuncture points can be proved by using electrical apparatus for 'detecting' them, but once again such claims usually do not stand up to serious scientific investigation. (I shall come back to this question later in more detail.)

Much the same applies to pulse diagnosis. This is an art rather than a science, but it is supposed to give factual information and it should therefore, in principle, be capable of objective verification: for example, by comparing the diagnoses of different physicians who have examined the same patients.

In Western medicine, the cardiologists of earlier days used to claim to be able to hear in the hearts of their patients all kinds of things which were not always audible to lesser mortals. The cardiologists in question naturally ascribed this to their own superior powers of discernment, but unfortunately when an instrument that could record the heart sounds was invented (the phonocardiograph), it usually failed to confirm the existence of the sounds described by the experts. Possibly the same will prove to be true of the Chinese pulses, although machines have been invented which purportedly provide objective evidence of the different types of pulse. Even if these findings are real, which is uncertain, we are still left with the problem of deciding what, if anything, the recorded pulse features signify. For reasons I have already explained it is difficult or impossible to make correlations between traditional Chinese medical diagnoses and those of modern medicine; but pulse diagnosis, of course, gives an answer in terms of traditional medicine.

Nevertheless, although the channels may not exist in an anatomical sense, this does not necessarily mean that they have no existence at all. We do not know how the idea of channels arose in the first place but one plausible guess is that they did so because patients do, in fact, sometimes report sensations that appear to support the notion. For example, some people have places on their skin which, when pressed or rubbed, cause similar feelings in quite remote areas. Rubbing the leg, for example, may cause an itch to appear in the face.

In some patients, inserting a needle in the right place actually gives rise to sensations travelling along the path of the appropriate channel. This can occur in people who do not know where the channels are supposed to be and who therefore cannot be thought to have suggested this pattern to themselves. The same is true of pain patterns in disease according to Macdonald (1984), who studied 52 consecutive patients suffering from various kinds of arthritis. Each patient was asked to sketch the pattern of his or her pain on a prepared outline drawing of the body. It turned out that there was a strong tendency for the patients' pains to follow the course of the channels.

It would be natural to conclude from such observations that there really are channels through which chi is propagated to give rise to the sensations in question, and this may be what happened in ancient China. To a modern anatomist, however, it is much more plausible (and probably more interesting) to regard such propagation of sensation as due to so far unknown connections within the nervous system. It seems likely, in fact, that the ancient Chinese physicians made a valid observation even if the theory they constructed to account for it no longer is tenable in the light of modern knowledge. Our own theories may well be seen to be equally untenable in time to come, of course, but for the moment they are the best we have and for most scientifically trained doctors it is psychologically impossibe to bring themselves to accept a mediaeval theoretical framework – and a Chinese one at that. If acupuncture is to be taken up seriously by Western doctors it is inevitable that they will reinterpret it in the light of their own concepts. This has the advantage, moreover, that new techniques, based on modern ideas, can be introduced into acupuncture. The Chinese themselves have shown great willingness to adopt such ideas and techniques; it is Western adherents of the traditional system who have usually shown themselves most rigid in maintaining the ancient theories and practices.

It might appear from this that I am dismissing the whole conceptual apparatus of ancient Chinese philosophy and science as worthless or irrelevant to ourselves. That would be an impossibly arrogant thing to do. On the contrary, I find Chinese thought an intensely fascinating study, and I believe that Taoism, in particular, with its reverence for Nature, is one of the most profound and wise philosophies that human beings have produced. Certainly it teaches many lessons that our civilisation would do well to learn before it is too late.

I hope, therefore, it will not seem arrogant if I say that, so far as *practical* acupuncture is concerned, it is best to approach the subject from a modern scientific point of view. And this may not be so much out of tune with the ancient Chinese tradition as might first appear, for Chinese medicine and science, though containing many elements that we might at first glance label as magical, were not metaphysical but on the contrary down to earth and essentially naturalistic. It should not be forgotten that, until the seventeeth century, Chinese science and technology were much in advance of anything the West could boast.

REFERENCES

Macdonald, A. (1984). *Acupuncture: From Chinese Art to Modern Medicine*, p. 42. George Allen and Unwin, London.

Needham, J. and Gwei-Djen, L. (1980). *Celestial Lancets: A History and Rationale of Acupuncture and Moxa*, p. 186. Cambridge University Press, Cambridge.

Chapter Two
SCIENTIFIC ACUPUNCTURE

Acupuncture first reached the attention of the West in the second half of the seventeenth century. The first European writer to mention the subject was a Dane, Jacob de Bondt, who was surgeon-general to the Dutch East India Company at Batavia. A more detailed account of the technique was given by a Dutchman, Willem ten Rhijne, who was also a physician in the service of the Dutch East India Company. He spent two years in Japan and 24 in Java. A number of other authors wrote accounts of acupuncture during the seventeenth century, and gradually a clearer picture began to appear. By the end of the century, it seems, acupuncture of a sort, and also moxibustion, were being practised quite widely in Western Europe.

In the early eighteenth century clinical interest in these techniques declined, though they still attracted scientific comment and several commentaries on them were written.

During the first half of the nineteenth century interest in acupuncture and moxibustion revived. However, the acupuncture was fairly elementary, and for the most part consisted simply in needling the painful area. Although a considerable amount of information about the channels and pulse diagnosis had reached the West, this made little impression on most Western doctors. The first book on acupuncture to appear in France was written by L. V. J. Berlioz, the father of the composer, in 1816. He obtained his best results, as might be expected, in rheumatism and arthritis and in muscle and joint stiffness after falls, but he also treated whooping cough and 'nervous fever'.

Another Frenchman, Le Chevalier Sarlandière, was the first to apply electric needles to the implanted needles. Writing in 1825 he reported cures in asthma, various forms of paralysis and migraine and rheumatism. Two other French physicians, Jules Coquet and his disciple T. M. Dantu, wrote extensively on acupuncture and described the treatment of many kinds of intractable pain including facial neuralgia. They sometimes left the needles in for as long as eight hours though they also reported near instantaneous relief of pain.

France was not the only European country to take up acupuncture at this time. Experiments using electrical stimulation were carried out in Italy. Acupuncture was adopted in Germany, but only to a limited extent. In England the first important advocate was J. M. Churchill, who published two books on acupuncture in 1821 and 1828. As usual, most of his successes were in what we would now call musculoskeletal disorders (rheumatism, sciatica, back pain, and so on), but he also, rather surprisingly, had good results in dropsy. He reported the teh chi effect (see p. 49) even though he did not know of its existence from Chinese writings.

Churchill's interest was rather slow to spread, but by the 1840s Leeds Infirmary had become a major acupuncture centre. By 1825 the practice of acupuncture had reached North America. By the middle of the century, however, Western interest in acupuncture was once more on the wane, being largely confined to charlatans.

In the last decades of the nineteenth century interest in acupuncture began yet another of its periodical revivals, and with some ups and downs the trend has has continued to the present time. In the 1920s and 1930s the French writer Soulié de Morant wrote some important books based directly on Chinese sources, while other influences came from Vietnam and Japan, both of which had long traditions of acupuncture.

Even so, it was not until President Nixon's visit to China in 1972 that acupuncture really came to the attention of the main body of the Western medical profession and, indeed, the public as a whole. What caught the general imagination was a most astonishing fact: the Chinese were apparently performing large numbers of surgical operations using acupuncture instead of conventional anaesthesia to prevent pain. Initial incredulity was dissipated when visiting Western doctors actually witnessed surgery carried out in this way. Admittedly, some remained sceptical, and it later emerged that the Chinese, in the grip of the Cultural Revolution, had indulged in exaggerated claims about the matter; even so, there certainly were some interesting phenomena to be explored. The consequence was that a number of researchers undertook studies to try to find out how acupuncture analgesia (rather than anaesthesia, for the patients remained conscious throughout) might be produced.

At about this time, meanwhile, a surprising discovery was made in the West. It was found that the body produces remarkable opium-like substances – the endorphins and enkephalins, as they were named – whose properties included the suppression of pain. This seemed to promise a rationale for the ability of acupuncture to reduce or abolish pain, for numerous experiments demonstrated that needling people (and animals) caused the release of these substances into the blood.

On the theoretical level, meanwhile, new ideas about the way in which pain impulses are transmitted in the nervous system were being introduced, largely through the work of Melzack and Wall (1982), and these too seemed to have relevance to acupuncture, which now began to seem not quite so outrageously improbable as it had done to most Western doctors and scientists only a short time before.

These developments led to a considerable increase of interest in acupuncture on the part of Western doctors, and although many continued to believe that the effects of acupuncture were wholly attributable to suggestion, research into the subject went on and gradually began to assume quite respectable proportions. At the same time, more and more Western doctors tried out acupuncture in practice and found that it worked. Little by little acupuncture was becoming respectable.

On the whole, however, Western doctors did not approach the subject from a traditional point of view but instead tried to reinterpret the phenomena within the framework of modern scientific understanding of how the body works. Hence there has grown up in the last 15 years or so a version of acupuncture which might be called physiological or scientific. This trend is anathema to purists who adhere to the traditional ideas, and undeniably there is a real danger of brashly scorning insights and observations of great value contained in the ancient tradition. Nevertheless, it seems inevitable that if acupuncture is ever to become as widely accepted and practised in the West as it deserves to be, such a melting down and recasting of the ancient knowledge is inevitable. Indeed, as I have already mentioned, the modern Chinese themselves do not seem to have any difficulty in absorbing new ways of looking at their ancient tradition: the use of acupuncture to prevent pain during operations, for example, is a new development. (There does, however, seem to be a long-standing practice in China of claiming that any new idea is actually an old one to be found somewhere or other in the ancient texts; such claims have been made for acupuncture analgesia as well as for other innovations adopted by the Chinese.)

In this book I am writing about *scientific* acupuncture, but I do not wish to imply by this term that it is anything like possible to explain all, or even most, of acupuncture effects in scientific terms. Far too little is known, either about acupuncture or about the nervous system, to support such an ambitious claim. I would say only that it is in principle possible to account for acupuncture effects in this way, but in the effort to do so we are likely to need to expand our ideas about physiology and neurology very considerably. What follows in this chapter, therefore, is certainly not intended to be a final statement but only to provide a crutch for the sceptical scientific intellect.

OUTLINE OF A SCIENTIFIC APPROACH

The scientific version of acupuncture is not based on the channels as real anatomical entities but instead regards acupuncture as working *via the nervous system*. As for acupuncture points, these are not thought of as entities necessarily fixed in location and possessing the properties described in the classic texts, but are reinterpreted in various ways that I shall discuss shortly. Pulse diagnosis is not used, and the concepts of disease are those generally accepted in Western medicine, though with a greater than usual emphasis on disorders of function.

Most Western theorising on acupuncture has been based on two things: the discovery of the endorphins and enkephalins and the 'gate theory' of Melzack and Wall (1982). I shall say a little about each of these and then mention some other ideas that also seem to be relevant.

1. Endorphins and enkephalins
These are members of a group of substances known collectively as the opioid neurotransmitters. They are so called because they resemble morphine in their ability to suppress pain and because they transmit impulses between nerve cells. Quite a family of these substances has now turned up. Their functions are by no means fully understood, but it has been suggested that they may explain the remarkable fact that people who suffer severe injuries, especially in conditions of great excitement (for example sportsmen or soldiers in battle), may feel no pain for some hours after the injury. It was therefore natural for people to suggest that these substances might be involved in acupuncture, and this idea has been supported to some extent by research. Acupuncture can cause their release. More precisely, if fast electrical stimulation (200Hz) is used one type of substance, met-enkephalin, is released, while if slow (manual or electrical) stimulation at about 2Hz is used a different substance, beta-endorphin, is released.

This research is certainly very interesting and possibly it does help to account for acupuncture analgesia during surgery. The release of these substances does not go on for very long, however, and it seems inadequate to account for the relief of pain lasting for days, weeks, or even permanently which can result from acupuncture.

On the other hand, the existence of these opioid neurotransmitters may explain one intriguing acupuncture effect. Some patients regularly feel euphoric, almost ecstatic, after acupuncture, and this state may last for several hours and be followed by drowsiness. People may describe the experience as like that of taking alcohol or hashish. The effect does not seem to be due to suggestion, for it occurs to patients who do not expect it and who are astonished by it. As a rule patients who react in this way prove to be good acupuncture subjects.

2. The 'gate' theory

Another clue to how acupuncture works may come from recent ways of looking at the way the nervous system processes pain. According to the older model, which goes back as far as Descartes for its ultimate inspiration, the nervous system is something like a telephone system. If, say, you tread on a drawing pin, a pain impulse travels up the nerves from your foot to your spinal cord and thence to the brain, where in some wholly mysterious way it reaches consciousness. This model is essentially a passive one, in that transmission of the painful stimulus is supposed to occur automatically provided the nervous pathways are intact. Melzack and Wall (1982), however, have pointed out that there are serious difficulties with this scheme. Sometimes a severe injury causes little pain. Conversely, a relatively trivial injury may at times cause agonising pain. Again, pain may persist for months or years after the injury that caused it has long ago healed completely.

Melzack and Wall (1982) believe that the older theories of pain cannot account for facts such as these. Instead they have proposed a new model, based on the idea that the brain does not just attend to single messages coming to it along specific nerve fibres but rather monitors *all* the information at its disposal before registering pain.

This is the basis of their 'gate' theory. To describe this in the sketchiest possible outline, what they suggest is that the spinal cord (and probably the brain as well) contain 'gates' which can open or close to allow pain impulses to pass to the brain or not, as the case may be (Fig. 2/1).

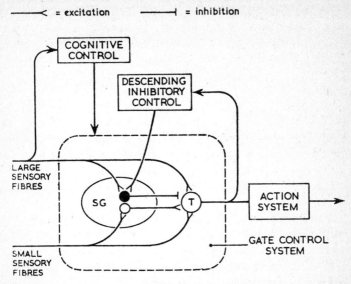

Fig. 2/1 The 'gate' theory of pain. SG = substantia gelatinosa;
T = transmission cells

Two kinds of nervous impulse are supposed to act on the
gates. Afferent impulses from the periphery can open or close
the gates, according to the type of nerve fibre involved (large
diameter fibres close the gates, small diameter fibres open
them). This provides an explanation for the fact that rubbing
the site of an injury may relieve the pain it causes, and it is also
relevant to acupuncture.

The second class of nervous impulse acting on the gates is
efferent or descending impulses from higher centres in the
brain, including those concerned with consciousness. Their
importance is that they help to explain how psychological
factors influence our perception of pain, and why patients who
are afraid of acupuncture or unwilling to have it seldom do well.
The main problem with the gate theory as an explanation for
acupuncture is once again the difficulty of accounting for the
long duration of pain relief that can be achieved. There are
ways round this problem, however. Melzack has suggested that

temporary relief of pain through acupuncture allows the patient to use the affected part more freely, and this leads to a more normal pattern of nervous impulses arriving in the brain. Repeated acupuncture would enhance this effect and so set up a 'virtuous circle' of progressive freedom from pain.

PAIN MEMORY

Fundamental to the idea of acupuncture I am advancing here is the notion that the central nervous system (brain and spinal cord) can retain a 'memory' of pain for long periods, even indefinitely, and that consequently there can exist 'causeless' pain.

To most patients, and indeed to many doctors, to suggest that pain can exist without a 'cause' in the ordinary sense of the word appears absurd. We are all familiar with the pain that arises from an acute injury, and it is natural to assume that when pain persists it must be due to some continuing injury. Yet there are facts that contradict this. For example, the brain itself cannot feel pain, but damage to the central core of the brain by a stroke can cause the so-called thalamic pain syndrome, in which the patient suffers severe chronic pain. This 'central pain', as it is called, is usually almost impossible to treat. Damage to the spinal cord can also cause intractable severe pain.

Another puzzle concerns the occurrence of pain in parts of the body which have lost their ability to feel anything or which even no longer exist. For example, the spinal cord may be cut, either accidentally or by the surgeon, in an attempt to control chronic pain. This paralyses the areas of the body that were supplied by the parts of the cord below the lesion and also abolishes all sensation in those areas, yet some patients continue to feel pain in parts of the body below the level of the injury. The explanation of the paradox, according to Melzack and Wall (1982a), is probably that the loss of sensory input from the lower parts of the body allows large numbers of cells in the cord to send abnormal volleys of impulses to the parts of the brain that are concerned with pain experience.

After amputation of a limb there is commonly a phantom limb; that is, the patient continues to feel that his limb is present. Phantoms, which may be of various kinds, are not necessarily undesirable; in fact, it seems that a phantom limb is necessary if an artificial limb is to be used, but phantoms may be excruciatingly painful. A patient may feel, for example, that his non-existent hand is tightly clenched, the finger nails digging agonisingly into his palm. The cause of these pains is not understood, but Melzack and Wall (1982b) suggest that they are again due to loss of the normal sensory input.

Persistent 'causeless' pain can follow many other kinds of injury. For example, motorcyclists who fall on their shoulders may tear out their brachial plexus – the sheaf of nerve fibres that emerges from the spinal cord in the lower neck to provide the nerve supply for the arm. This injury results in a paralysed arm lacking normal sensation, but the patient may nevertheless experience agonising pain the the arm.

It is not only major injuries that give rise to intractable pain. Sometimes persistent pain may follow an apparently trivial injury, such as a bruise, a thorn prick, or (as happened to a friend of mine) a poke in the eye from the corner of a card.

The importance of pain memory
It might seem that pain of the kind I have just described is a fortunately rare and exceptional event. Probably, however, it is really very common. It seems quite possible that many kinds of chronic pain, perhaps most, are due to *changes within the central nervous system*. Unfortunately we do not know in detail what these changes may be, but there is a growing belief among researchers into pain and its treatment that something of this kind occurs. Those of us who are not experts in the field may perhaps be content with a grossly simplified picture. We may think of chronic pain as due to the persistence of abnormal patterns of nerve cell activity in the brain or spinal cord, which may persist for long periods. They may be analogous to the 'loops' that sometimes occur in computer programmes, or to a persistent eddy in a stream.

This idea has important practical consequences. Back pain

and sciatica, for example, may be due to a lumbar disc that has protruded and compressed the nerve roots (the so-called slipped disc). But what actually causes the pain in such cases? The usual explanation is that the disc irritates the nerve and makes it send volleys of 'pain impulses' into the spinal cord. An alternative theory, however, is that it is *loss* of incoming impulses that causes nerve cells in the spinal cord to fire spontaneously and abnormally and so give rise to pain. This idea may explain why operation to remove the damaged disc does not always abolish the pain.

Perhaps there is also an explanation here for the long-lasting pain that sometimes follows trivial injuries. It may be that such injuries can sometimes, for unknown reasons, 'set' the nervous system in a particular mode that gives rise to pain. We could picture the central nervous system as containing pain control dials, something like those on thermostats, which can be set to a particular value by nerve impulses arriving from outside. In certain circumstances a dial may be turned to a low setting, at which it puts the pain mechanisms into constant activity. And unless it is re-set to a higher value the pain will continue indefinitely, perhaps for the remainder of that patient's life. This explains why some unfortunate patients may be subjected to repeated surgical operations to relieve persistent unexplained back or abdominal pain, for example. None of these does any good, and eventually the patients are usually labelled as neurotic, for want of a better explanation for their pain.

Treating pain memory
If the theory I have just outlined is right – and there is increasing evidence that it is, at least in many cases of chronic pain – it follows that the treatment must be directed, not at the site of the original injury, but at the nervous system. The aim of treatment, in fact, must be to re-set the 'pain thermostat'.

There are many ways of trying to do this. Sometimes blocking the sympathetic nervous system in the region helps dramatically, for reasons that are not fully understood. Sometimes electrical stimulation is applied directly to the spinal cord, via implanted electrodes. And there are many other sophisticated techniques involving the use of surgery or drugs.

In addition to these, however, there are also relatively simple physical techniques, some of which are probably as old as mankind. They include massage, manipulation, application of heat or cold, and electrical stimulation. All these are really more or less sophisticated developments of the quite instinctive tendency we all possess to scratch an itch, stretch a stiff back or limb, or rub a place that hurts. (I can still remember making the interesting scientific discovery, at the age of 5, that rubbing my skin after I had been slapped significantly diminished the pain.)

Acupuncture, I suggest, should be looked upon as one physical method among others for re-setting the pain thermostats. Like the other methods, it has its advantages and disadvantages, but what they all have in common is that they are techniques for sending nerve impulses into the brain and spinal cord.

We can now begin to make at least some sense of the hitherto totally mysterious fact that merely putting a needle briefly into a patient can relieve her pain for long periods or even permanently. Just as a trivial injury can sometimes turn on a pain thermostat and cause pain that persists for years or even a lifetime, so inserting a needle can sometimes have the opposite effect.

Admittedly it is not yet possible to explain in detail how this occurs. Clinical experience suggests, however, that what is needed is to recreate the stimulus that originally gave rise to the pain. Possibly this occurs when endorphins are released. It seems that these substances may be able to re-set the nerve cells in a particular mode, and so abolish pain. If so, this would provide an elegant explanation for the long-term effects of acupuncture.

ACUPUNCTURE POINTS: TRIGGER POINTS: MOTOR POINTS

The phenomenon of *referred pain* is very important in medicine generally and in acupuncture in particular. It has long been recognised that patients may feel pain at a site remote from the scene of injury or disease. The pain of heart disease – angina pectoris – may radiate down the left arm and, exceptionally, may be felt at only one place, such as the wrist. The pain of acute appendicitis is traditionally referred to a site in the lower right quadrant of the abdomen, known as McBurney's point. The occurrence of such patterns of referred pain is well known and is used in diagnosis.

What is less well known, however, is the fact that there also exist relatively small areas which, when pressed with the fingers or pierced with a needle, cause pain to be felt in a different, sometimes remote, area or organ of the body. The existence of these *trigger points* (TPs), as they are called, is almost neglected by mainstream scientific medicine. Most Western medical textbooks either ignore the whole subject completely or else refer to it by one or other of a large number of confusing terms, such as fibrositis, muscular rheumatism, or myalgia. Yet TPs are easy to find if one looks for them.

For example, patients suffering from angina pectoris mostly show a more or less standard pattern of TPs in the chest and shoulders. Pressure on these TPs often produces intense pain lasting for hours. What is particularly interesting, however, is that normal people also have such TPs, which likewise give rise to pain when pressed though it is less severe and prolonged.

Even more surprising is the fact that injecting a local anaesthetic into the TP abolishes not only the TP itself, as one might expect, but often the referred pain as well. What this suggests is that the pain experienced in many kinds of disease is a 'summation' pain.

For instance, it can be notoriously difficult to decide whether a given patient's chest pain is coming from her heart or from her oesophagus. Sometimes investigations show that there is some inflammation of the lower end of the oesophagus, and when this is treated the pain vanishes. Does this prove that the pain was coming from her oesophagus and not her heart? Not necessarily. Sometimes, it seems, there is disease in *both* organs, but neither by itself gives rise to enough disturbance to register as pain. The combination of the two, however, does cause pain. If one of the two organs is now treated, the pain disappears even though the other organ is still diseased.

The most systematic and exhaustive study of TPs in Western scientific literature has been made by two American doctors, J. G. Travell and D. G. Simons (see Bibliography). They define myofascial TPs as loci of hyper-irritability in muscles or their associated connective tissue which, when compressed, are locally tender and which may give rise to referred pain, referred tenderness, or remote autonomic phenomena.

Almost everyone has at least a few *latent* TPs; for example, G21, in the upper trapezius muscle at the midpoint of the shoulder, is tender on pressure in most people. *Active* TPs are tender spontaneously. Both active and latent TPs can, when stimulated, give rise to referred pain and other remote effects.

Not much is known about what TPs actually are. It has been suggested that they are localised collections of fluid (oedema), localised muscle spasm or arterio-venous shunts. In many cases they can come and go surprisingly rapidly, their number and activity changing almost from moment to moment. On the other hand, they can also be very persistent, lasting in some cases for many years.

It seems that they can arise in a variety of ways: trauma (for example a sudden muscular strain), chilling and infections of various kinds seem to cause them, and so does psychological stress. But it also seems that what is abnormal is often not the presence of the TP *per se* but rather its degree of activity. Activity may develop suddenly or gradually. As a TP becomes more active it begins to be more tender when pressed and may now also be associated with a pattern of referred pain. If the degree of activity rises still further the TP may become painful spontaneously, even without being pressed, and the referred pain may be present continuously.

TPs can also give rise to symptoms other than pain, including weakness, localised sweating, excessive tear formation, dizziness, tinnitus and disorders of various internal organs. For this reason, the study and treatment of TPs requires a knowledge of general medicine.

The number of TPs is very variable. There may be only one or two, or there may be scores. Individual patients vary greatly in their liability to produce TPs. Most surveys have shown them to be commoner in women than in men. The prevalence of active TPs increases throughout life up to middle age, after which it tends to decline, perhaps owing to reduced physical activity, although part of the stiffness found in most old people may be due to latent TPs.

In the context of acupuncture it is natural to ask to what extent TPs can be correlated with acupuncture points. And the answer seems to be that to a large extent they can be so correlated. In 1977 Melzack and two colleagues studied this question and concluded that every TP reported in Western literature has a corresponding acupuncture point. Moreover, in 71 per cent of cases there is a close correspondence between the patterns of pain associated with the two kinds of point. On the basis of this study they concluded that TPs and acupuncture points for pain are different descriptions of the same phenomenon.

A number of Western doctors have described methods of treating symptoms associated with TPs. Simple pressure is quite effective (acupressure); the TP is pressed so as to cause discomfort but not severe pain, and as the sensation diminishes the pressure is increased to maintain the same level of discomfort; this process is continued for 2 or 3 minutes. Travell and Simons favour relaxing the affected muscle by means of a cooling spray and then stretching it, though they also use an injection technique. Injection has been used by a number of other people: corticosteroids, local anaesthetics and plain saline have been used chiefly, though a few therapists have taken the logical next step of just putting in a needle, without injecting anything. Those who have done so have nearly always found that it worked as well, or almost as well, as injecting something.

As a variant on the TP theme, some researchers have concentrated on *muscle motor points*. A motor point (or zone) is that region of the muscle where the main motor nerve enters and supplies it; usually, though not always, the motor point is situated in or near the mid-zone of the muscle. There is not necessarily a conflict between this idea and that of TPs, since TPs and motor points frequently coincide. Not all TPs, however, are found in the motor points of muscles; they may also occur, for example, at the junction between muscle and tendon, over superficial nerve plexuses and in other places.

A SIMPLIFIED VERSION OF ACUPUNCTURE

On the basis of the ideas I have discussed in this chapter it becomes possible, I believe, to put forward a simple scheme for understanding what one is doing when one practises acupuncture. It is, no doubt, over-simple, but it has the merit of providing a practical framework within which it is possible to devise treatments that are innovative as well as effective.

There are, I suggest, four main kinds of acupuncture, each with its own characteristics and range of applications: local acupuncture, trigger point acupuncture, segmental acupuncture and generalised acupuncture.

1. Local acupuncture

This is the simplest form of all and consists merely in needling the painful area itself. Some purists refuse to allow this form of treatment the name of acupuncture, an attitude which seems to me to be hairsplitting, especially in view of the fact that the method is described in Chinese texts as far back as the seventh century AD.

2. Trigger point acupuncture

This is the commonest type of acupuncture and is used in a wide range of musculoskeletal disorders, including muscular rheumatism and arthritis of various kinds. It consists, as the name implies, in searching for and treating (by needling) some or all of the TPs that are found. These may or may not coincide with classic acupuncture points, but in any case it is the presence of the TP, rather than the textbook situation of any relevant acupuncture point, that decides where the needle shall be inserted.

3. Segmental acupuncture

In this type of acupuncture the needles are inserted on the basis of the known distribution of dermatomes, myotomes, or sclerotomes, that is, within the relevant spinal segment or segments. It may not matter much exactly where the needles are inserted within this fairly broad region. The principal application of this treatment is to periosteal acupuncture, which I shall discuss in a later chapter. Ear acupuncture could perhaps be considered as a special form of this type of acupuncture.

4. Generalised acupuncture

This form is typically used in treating a generalised disorder, such as an allergy or a psychological problem. In such cases TPs are of lesser significance and the aim of treatment is to try to stimulate a general reaction. Sometimes it may not seem to matter very much where the needles are inserted for this purpose, but certain areas do seem to cause more reaction than others. The hands and feet are particularly useful in this way, and commonly used points are 'Liver 3' in the foot and 'Large Intestine 4' in the hand, probably because they are situated in areas that are abundantly supplied with nerves and which consequently give rise to a strong stimulus when needled.

It will be seen that this scheme makes no mention of classical acupuncture points. This omission is deliberate and reflects my own uncertainty about the existence of these things, an uncertainty I seem to share with many other doctors practising scientific acupuncture. There is no doubt that many, in fact most, acupuncture points can be related to commonly encountered TPs, and probably it is satisfactory to regard TPs and acupuncture points as the same thing in so far as the treatment of painful disorders is concerned. What is still, I think, uncertain is whether there are specific points which, when stimulated, have specific effects that cannot be obtained by stimulating other points. For example, does S36 have the property of influencing the immune system, as it is sometimes said to do? I do not think we have the evidence to decide such questions one way or the other.

To complicate matters still further, it has to be remembered that in some cases it may make little difference where the needles are inserted. To many critics this statement is equivalent to an admission that acupuncture is merely a placebo treatment, but the real state of affairs is a good deal less simple.

Like any other form of treatment, acupuncture has a considerable placebo effect. In addition, however, there appears to be an effect due to needling, regardless of the exact site at which it is performed. This phenomenon has been called 'diffuse noxious inhibitory control'. A painful input from anywhere in the body, provided it is strong enough, may abolish a pre-existing pain, at least temporarily. This fact has important consequences for research in acupuncture. Studies (see Chapter 10) have been made to compare 'real' with 'sham' acupuncture (that is, needling done at the 'correct' sites and needling done at random sites), but the phenomenon of diffuse noxious inhibitory control makes them very difficult to evaluate, and many medical acupuncturists feel that 'sham' acupuncture of this kind is not a valid placebo for research purposes.

There is a curious paradox here which should be mentioned. Doctors often put needles into patients for reasons not connected directly with treatment; to take blood samples, for instance, or to perform electromyograms. Needling patients for these purposes does not usually relieve pain, yet it should do, at least at times, if the concept of diffuse noxious inhibitory control is correct. So why does it not do so?

The answer seems to be that the nervous system has to be 'primed', as it were, for treatment: the patient must be *expecting* to be treated. Notice that this does not mean that she should necessarily believe in the treatment; indeed, I often find that my best results are in patients who confess later that they did not think acupuncture would work. What matters is that the patient should regard the setting as one in which treatment is to be given and should be willing for this to occur. For this reason it is important to give adequate time to explaining what is going to happen and making sure that the patient understands and is willing to be treated.

ACUPUNCTURE IN NON-PAINFUL DISORDERS

Acupuncture as a treatment for non-painful disorders receives rather little attention in Western medical literature, most writers seeming to prefer to concentrate on pain, acute or chronic. This appears to be due to a reluctance to stray too far from the known; psychologically the idea of using acupuncture to treat pain is just about acceptable, at least for some doctors, but to go on to using it for non-painful disorders somehow involves a suspension of disbelief that many find too difficult. Yet most people who use acupuncture a lot find that it works very well for a number of non-painful disorders, indeed some of its most interesting applications are to be found here. There are in fact quite respectable reasons for believing that acupuncture could be useful in such cases.

Given that acupuncture stimulates release of endorphins, it is becoming increasingly clear that these substances have far-reaching effects not confined to pain suppression. They are neurotransmitters – messengers between nerve cells. Moreover, the endorphin molecules are fragments of a larger molecule produced by the pituitary gland, beta-lipotropin, which splits up to produce endorphin and adrenocorticotrophic hormone (ACTH). It is thus entirely reasonable to suppose that acupuncture might affect various aspects of hormone secretion via the hypothalamus.

There may also be effects on the immune system. The immune system is partly under nervous control, and there is therefore nothing inherently improbable in the notion that stimulating nerve rich areas of the body could modify, say, resistance to infection. Of course, to say that such effects are conceivable is not to prove that they occur. To demonstrate that will take decades of research and much theoretical work, but at least the idea is not self-evidently absurd.

Nevertheless, the limitations of acupuncture must be remembered. Even in ancient China it was never a complete system of medicine and this is certainly true today. It is a valuable treatment and in a number of circumstances it is the best available, but it is not suitable for every problem by any means. It should, in fact, be thought of as part of general medicine.

REFERENCES

Melzack, R., Stillwell, D. M. and Fox, E. J. (1977). Trigger points and acupuncture points for gain: correlations and implications. *Pain*, 3, 3–23.

Melzack, R. and Wall, P. (1982). *The Challenge of Pain*. Penguin Books, Harmondsworth.

ibid. (1982a). pp. 84–6.

ibid. (1982b). pp. 76–84.

Chapter Three
LEARNING ACUPUNCTURE

WHO SHOULD LEARN?

In many countries today the practice of acupuncture is strictly regulated. In Britain, however, anyone at all may practise acupuncture and call himself or herself an acupuncturist. There are no formally recognised training courses or qualifications in acupuncture, and there is nothing to stop anyone who wishes to do so from placing an advertisement in the local paper and starting to practise even if he cannot tell an acupuncture needle from a knitting needle. (Indeed, I heard recently of an unemployed welder who did just that.)

At a more serious level, there are schools of traditional Chinese acupuncture that accept both doctors and lay people as students. The courses at these establishments last several years and at the end of the course successful students receive a diploma. Such diplomas, however, have no status in law and there is no easy way for a would-be patient (or her doctor) to know what sort of training the diploma holder has undergone.

So far as patients are concerned, this situation is obviously unsatisfactory. People who want to have acupuncture treatment must make up their own minds about whom to consult, often on inadequate evidence, and unless their own general practitioner happens to practise acupuncture himself or to know about the subject, which is possible but unlikely, they will find it difficult to obtain reliable guidance. On the whole the freedom to practise various forms of alternative medicine which we enjoy in this country is good, but in the case of acupuncture there are some special problems, since the treatment is potentially hazardous. It consists, after all, in sticking needles into people, with all the risks that this entails, so it is clearly essential that the acupuncturist should at least know anatomy and be familiar with proper methods of sterilisation. This is one good reason for entrusting oneself only to doctors. Another is that non-medical acupuncturists cannot be assumed to be capable of recognising symptoms that may point to serious underlying disease. For example, they may well not realise that the recent onset of constipation in a previously healthy middle-aged man or woman is, by itself, a symptom demanding immediate investigation to exclude cancer of the intestine. They also may not be aware that acupuncture can mask serious underlying diseases by removing its symptoms temporarily. This was confirmed by a study, carried out not long ago at the National Hospital for Nervous Diseases, in which it was found that acupuncture could temporarily relieve headache caused by brain tumour.

In some cases, of course, the risks are not so great. If a patient has suffered from arthritis for years there is no danger of masking underlying disease, and she would be safe, from this point of view, in attending an acupuncturist who was not medically qualified, although of course the proviso about the dangers of acupuncture itself would still apply.

In recent years a number of physiotherapists have started to practise acupuncture, regarding it as a natural extension of their own work on the musculoskeletal system. At some hospitals where acupuncture is used it is the physiotherapists who normally carry out the treatment at the request of the consultant in charge.

It is certainly true that the actual performance of acupuncture is essentially a practical affair, requiring an ability to use one's hands effectively to detect TPs and insert the needles skilfully, and these are practices that physiotherapists might well be able to acquire, probably more quickly than some doctors. There thus seems to be a reasonable case to be made for acupuncture to be carried out by suitably trained physiotherapists in co-operation with the doctor who is in overall charge of the patient's treatment.

Whether it is desirable for physiotherapists to treat patients entirely on their own, without reference to a doctor at all, is another question. If the diagnosis is certain (for example, in cases of long-standing arthritis), there seems no reason why they should not. However, the basis of the approach I am using in this book is that *acupuncture is part of general medicine* and if this idea is accepted it follows that the right person to perform it will in most cases be a doctor.

There are several reasons for this. The decision to use acupuncture in a given case is seldom an entirely simple one. The patient has to want to be treated in this way, or at least not to be unwilling, but that is only the beginning. The therapist must consider other factors: the likelihood of success, the advantages and disadvantages of acupuncture compared with orthodox treatment, and the interrelationship of acupuncture with any treatment that the patient may be having for other diseases, for example. These are essentially medical questions.

There also are other advantages if acupuncture is practised by a doctor. In many cases patients present strange combinations of symptoms that may have led to their being referred to specialist after specialist, without result. A doctor who is familiar with acupuncture can review the patient's history and conclude that acupuncture is worth trying. The results in such cases are sometimes outstandingly good, but it is these problems, in particular, which demand a wide knowledge of clinical medicine. Acupuncture may not be the right treatment at all, but a consultation with a doctor who practises acupuncture provides a fresh medical opinion that may produce a new idea in *orthodox* treatment.

A criticism that one sometimes hears from enthusiasts for traditional acupuncture concerns the adequacy of the acupuncture training undergone by many Western doctors. How, it is asked, can a doctor acquire, in a single week or perhaps even a weekend, all the knowledge that a traditionalist absorbs over several years? The answer, plainly, is that it cannot be done. To master all the conceptual intricacies of the traditional system, let alone acquire the skills needed for pulse diagnosis, inevitably requires years of study. But it is by no means clear that this knowledge can be acquired *at all* in the West, by people lacking a knowledge of the Chinese language; more probably it would be necessary to spend a number of years in China, studying at the feet of acknowledged masters, and to learn enough Chinese to read the authentic texts. Needless to say, very few Westerners have been able to do this.

Scientific acupuncture, however, is another matter. Traditionalists may say that this is not 'real' acupuncture, but whatever one chooses to call it, it works. Sometimes we are told that the traditional method works better, but claims that the reverse is true are also made; in the absence of properly designed comparative trials this is a sterile controversy. Certainly one advantage of the modern physiological approach is that it is very flexible, able to incorporate new ideas derived from other sources as they arise. It seems to me self-evident that the sensible course is to make use of the best things in both schools of acupuncture, traditional and modern. As I have already mentioned, the present-day Chinese themselves appear to be very flexible in their approach.

In any case, experience over a number of years has shown that it is, in fact, perfectly possible to teach physiological acupuncture effectively *to doctors* in as short a time as a weekend. This is because doctors already possess the knowledge of anatomy, physiology and pathology that is the basis for acupuncture. This is not to say that a weekend is enough to make a doctor into a fully competent acupuncturist; of course it is not, but it does provide a foundation on which the doctor can build.

For doctors there are courses of various kinds. Most are short (a week or less), though some are longer and are spread out over a number of months at weekends. Some of these courses are in scientific acupuncture, some are traditional, and others are in various forms of electro-acupuncture.

For doctors interested in acupuncture there exists a society, the British Medical Acupuncture Society (BMAS), which holds meetings two or three times a year and acts as a focus for those

interested in the subject. Although the BMAS provides guidelines for courses run by its members, these are advisory only. The
BMAS does not hold examinations or issue a diploma and
doctors do not have to be members of the BMAS in order to
practise acupuncture.

HOW TO LEARN ACUPUNCTURE

A range of knowledge is required for success in acupuncture. A
thorough knowledge of modern anatomy, physiology and medicine is essential as a starting point. Next, the student needs to
become familiar with the concepts outlined in Chapters 1 and 2;
these provide the theoretical framework within which it is possible to make some kind of sense of acupuncture. This theoretical
knowledge can be obtained from books; what cannot be so
obtained is *practical* skill in examining patients for TPs and in
using the needles.

The ideal way of teaching this practical knowledge would be by
an 'apprenticeship' system, in which the student would spend
some weeks or months working with a skilled acupuncturist.
Such a prolonged learning period is however out of the question
for most doctors, who have their usual work to attend to.
Moreover, it is not strictly necessary because the essentials of
acupuncture practice are actually surprisingly simple and can
easily be demonstrated to doctors in a couple of days. After this it
is a matter of the doctor's putting them into practice and developing the manual skills on which successful acupuncture largely
depends. These skills are similar, though not identical, to those
required for examining abdomens, taking blood samples, and so
on, which a doctor necessarily acquires during his or her orthodox training. They are thus not wholly new challenges and the
skills usually do not take long to develop, though admittedly
individuals do vary in their innate manual dexterity, and there
will always be some doctors who are unsuited to practise acupuncture, just as there are some who are unsuited to be surgeons.

Once the essentials have been grasped it is up to the doctor to
extend his skill by using the technique and developing his ability.
Dr Felix Mann has said that a doctor will not become a good

acupuncturist unless he eventually reaches the stage of practising acupuncture for at least 20 per cent of his time, and I think this is probably a fair statement, although it does not follow that he cannot do any good to his patients before reaching this level of expertise. On the contrary, I cannot emphasise enough that *acupuncture is essentially simple*, and a doctor who has grasped the essentials will begin to get good results right from the beginning. What comes with time and experience is mainly the ability to apply acupuncture to new kinds of problems and, ultimately, to devise new kinds of treatment. As for further study, this is much more a question of reading books and papers on related subjects such as neurology, rheumatology and physical medicine rather than acupuncture books *per se*, since these tend to be repetitive and provide few new ideas.

Because modern acupuncture is still a very new and rapidly developing subject, it makes little sense, in my view, to speak about advanced courses in acupuncture. The phrase 'advanced acupuncture' implies that there exists an established body of esoteric knowledge needing long study for its acquisition; but this is simply not so, at least so far as physiological acupuncture is concerned. The whole subject is indeed so new that there is very little firm knowledge about it, and any pronouncements (including my own, of course) can only be an expression of personal opinion. Over-ambitious claims that this or that method of practising acupuncture is the best cannot be substantiated, first because we know far too little about how acupuncture really works, and second because comparative trials of different forms of treatment have not been made. In the absence of firm evidence the temptation to dogmatism is considerable, but it ought to be resisted.

The best way for a doctor already practising acupuncture to extend his knowledge is, apart from reading, to attend acupuncture meetings, formal or informal, and to talk to colleagues. Comparing notes in this way is a most valuable method of learning, and in my experience is often more fruitful than listening to set lectures. There are now numerous acupuncture meetings each year, both in this country and abroad, and it is always open to a group of doctors practising acupuncture in a particular locality to get together informally at intervals to discuss their experiences.

In summary, learning scientific acupuncture requires, for a doctor, the following steps.

1. Attend a course taught by a competent tutor.
2. Start to treat patients and gradually extend the range of practice as skill and confidence develop.
3. Read *around* the subect (not usually books on acupuncture *per se*).
4. Attend follow-up meetings and compare the experiences of other doctors practising acupuncture.

THE CONTENT OF COURSES

There are now over a dozen acupuncture courses for doctors being held at various times and places in this country throughout the year. The content of these courses varies considerably. One or two teach traditional acupuncture but the majority do not. Some place a lot of emphasis on the use of electrical apparatus while others, including my own, are mainly concerned with manual acupuncture. There are also courses devoted to special forms of acupuncture such as auriculo-therapy.

The content of courses is thus quite individual and reflects the interests and views of their organisers, but the BMAS has made certain recommendations about what every course should contain. For example, courses in traditional Chinese medicine should contain an outline of the scientific evidence for acupuncture, and conversely courses in scientific acupuncture should provide a brief introduction to the traditional concepts and terminology.

One reason why the content of courses varies quite a bit is that the different tutors and course organisers work in differing kinds of practice. Some are in general practice, some in private practice, and some, like myself, work mainly in hospitals. All these doctors necessarily see rather different types of patient. Perhaps the biggest difference is between the full-time and part-time practice of acupuncture. Each has its advantages and disadvantages. Full-time acupuncturists, of whom there are a few, treat a wide range of symptoms and diseases, which gives them good experience of acupuncture, but acupuncture is by no means suitable for treating everything, so full-time acupuncture tends to limit practitioners clinically.

On the other hand, if one practises acupuncture as part of general medicine there is a temptation to limit its application to those things for which one knows it does well and not to branch out into unknown territory. The best solution for this problem is to make a deliberate effort to extend one's range from time to time.

Whatever the bias of a particular course, traditional or physiological, there are certain basic things it should contain. These include instruction in the techniques of needling, and the view of most tutors, myself included, is that no one should practise acupuncture without direct experience of the typical needle sensation. This means that all the course participants needle each other. Much of the rest of the time is taken up with explaining and demonstrating how to examine patients for TPs and how and when to use the various kinds of treatment.

The aim of a course, I believe, should be to teach principles rather than to give students lists of 'points' to use (the so-called cook book approach). If acupuncture is taught in the way I advocate, doctors can begin to apply it on their own and to integrate it with what they already know and do.

USEFUL ADDRESS

The British Medical Acupuncture Society
67–69 Chancery Lane
London WC2A 1AF

Chapter Four
ACUPUNCTURE TOOLS AND THEIR USE

There are probably many similarities between acupuncture on the one hand and other forms of physical treatment such as manipulation, massage, and, of course, the absurdly named 'acupressure' on the other, since all are methods of applying local stimulation. However, acupuncture, by definition, implies the use of needles, so in describing the practical aspects of the techniques the first thing to discuss is the needles.

NEEDLES (Fig. 4/1)

It is possible to use ordinary injection needles for acupuncture but these have two disadvantages; they possess a sharp cutting edge and so are more likely to cause tissue damage or bleeding, and for some reason it seems to be more difficult to obtain teh chi (see p. 49) with them. It is also possible that, being hollow, they are more liable to introduce infection. They do, however, have two advantages: they are sterile and they are stiffer than acupuncture needles, which makes them easier to insert. For routine purposes, nevertheless, proper acupuncture needles are preferable.

Modern acupuncture needles are made from various substances, including gold and silver. Some writers on acupuncture believe that gold or silver needles possess special properties, but there is no good scientific evidence for this; stainless steel needles are equally satisfactory and are cheaper.

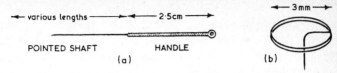

Fig. 4/1 (a) conventional acupuncture needle; (b) press needle

The Chinese needles in common use have two sections: a pointed shaft and a handle (Fig. 4/1a). The handle is usually made of fine wire wound round the upper part of the shaft. It is possible to buy needles with steel shafts and silver wire handles, but there is no advantage in this and in fact the silver handles are less satisfactory than the steel ones.

Needles come in various thicknesses, denoted by a gauge number, and in different lengths. The most generally useful size is 30mm 30 gauge, but routine acupuncture also requires longer needles on occasion; these are commonly 50mm 28 gauge. (The longer needles are thicker to make them easier to manipulate.) The Chinese sometimes use still longer needles but Western acupuncturists seldom do so. Shorter needles (15mm) are often used by those who practise ear acupuncture, though 30mm needles can also be used for this purpose.

Other types of needle also exist. There are *press needles* (Fig. 4/1b), something like a small drawing pin, that may be inserted in the ear and left in place for some days. Japanese acupuncturists favour extremely fine needles, hardly thicker than a hair, which have to be inserted with an introducer. Recently, there has been a vogue for pre-sterilised needles; these are a good idea in principle, but are too expensive for people who do a lot of acupuncture; they also may be of rather poor quality. Yet another instrument is the 'plum blossom hammer', which is a hammer containing several short needles fixed in its face; it is used to provide superficial stimulation over a wide area.

When first starting to practise acupuncture, it would probably be sufficient to buy, say, 10 or 20 50mm and 40 or 50 30mm needles.

CLEANING AND STERILISATION

The needles should be cleaned after use, before they are sterilised; this is to remove any traces of blood left from the patient as well as skin debris from the fingers of the acupuncturist. The needles can be cleaned with a cloth or tissue, though if many are in use it is quicker, as well as more effective, to use a small ultrasonic cleaner.

Sterilisation is, of course, vital. It must be adequate not merely to kill any bacteria that may have contaminated the needles but also to destroy viruses, especially those causing hepatitis and the acquired immune deficiency syndrome (AIDS). Although in the past makeshift methods might have been adequate, this is no longer true today and the only satisfactory standard is that appropriate for surgical instruments. In practice, this means autoclaving. Ideally this should be done in a hospital central sterilising department, but if this is not possible a small steriliser is an acceptable alternative. Doctors can obtain advice on these essential matters from the Infection Control Officer in their local district.

USING THE TOOLS

1. Inserting the needle (Fig. 4/2)
This skill cannot be learned from books but requires personal instruction and practice for its acquisition. It is essential that the needle be inserted as quickly and painlessly as possible, even though a certain amount of pain is sometimes inevitable. Unnecessary pain may interfere with the patient's response to treatment and is certainly liable to diminish her enthusiasm for this form of therapy.

Doctors and others who are familiar with giving injections are likely to be surprised by the difficulty they may encounter in inserting an acupuncture needle. This is because these needles are flexible and therefore have to be supported while being inserted. It is no use holding an acupuncture needle by the handle for this purpose; rather the mid-point of the shaft should be squeezed firmly between index finger and thumb of the right

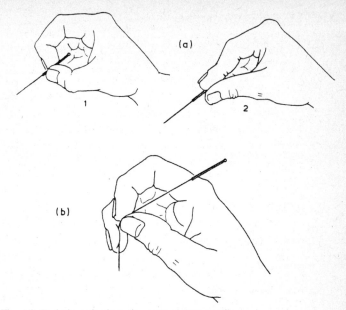

Fig. 4/2 Technique for inserting acupuncture needles

hand (Fig. 4/2a) (assuming a right-handed acupuncturist) while the patient's skin is stretched with the left hand so as to make it taut. The needle is then pushed forward by a quick movement of the finger and thumb. It should if at all possible penetrate the full depth of the skin in one action. If the point remains within the skin instead of passing through it (usually the result of an over-timid thrust) the result is considerable pain for the patient.

Some people have remarkably tough skins, which can present a considerable obstacle to the relatively blunt point of an acupuncture needle. In such cases it may be easier to penetrate the skin if this is done with several quick short pushes. This technique is particularly useful in places, such as the neck, where the skin may be lax. An alternative technique, described in some of the Chinese texts, is to 'drill' the needle through the skin with a twisting action.

The foregoing remarks apply particularly to 30mm needles. The 50mm needles are more difficult to insert, being more flexible. I find that the best way of using these is to hold them between the thumb and two fingers of the right hand and to bend them nearly to a right angle, so that perhaps half an inch of the shaft projects beyond the lowest finger (Fig. 4/2b).

People who find these manoeuvres difficult can use an introducer, which is simply a sterile tube that is placed over the site to be needled; the needle is inserted in the tube and tapped home. This technique is perfectly satisfactory but is seldom used by people who do a lot of acupuncture; of course, it adds considerably to the amount of sterilising.

2. Stimulation

After the needle is inserted a short pause should be allowed to assess the effect on the patient. There is normally a moment's pain as the needle goes through the skin but this should pass off quickly; if not, the needle should be taken out and reinserted a few millimetres away. Throughout, the patient's face should be carefully watched to assess her response and she should be asked repeatedly about what she is feeling.

If there is no particular effect after the initial insertion of the needle, stimulation may begin. The usual method of stimulating is by *twirling* the needle. This twirling may be done gently or strongly, according to the patient's response. Another method of stimulating the needle is what the Chinese call 'pecking' – that is, moving the needle up and down. This technique is used particularly for stimulating the periosteum.

One of the unresolved questions in acupuncture is whether it is necessary to stimulate at all. Some experienced acupuncturists believe that it is enough simply to insert the needle and leave it for a few minutes, without doing anything further; others, in contrast, find that nothing happens unless some stimulation is given. (To complicate matters still further, some people believe that the whole effect is produced within the first few seconds after the needle is inserted, because the nervous system adapts so quickly to the stimulus.) My own feeling is that in most cases it is necessary to give at least a brief twirl to the needle to start a reaction, although there are exceptions.

EFFECTS OF ACUPUNCTURE

Once the needle is inserted, a number of things may happen.

1. Local effects

(a) The *acupuncturist* may feel a resistance to twirling the needle. This may occur in two ways. It may be due to elastic fibres in the skin gripping the needle, in which case it is not significant, or it may be due to 'muscle grasp'. This phenomenon is not completely understood but is thought to be a localised muscle spasm caused by reflex activity. It is the basis of teh chi as experienced by the acupuncturist. It can be surprisingly strong and may make it difficult or impossible to withdraw the needle. Usually it will die away within a few minutes, after which the needle can be withdrawn easily, but if not it can be abolished by inserting a second needle at a little distance from the first.

(b) The *patient* may, as already noted, feel a sharp pain at the moment the needle is inserted, but this should pass off quickly. There may then ensue a variety of sensations which are usually difficult for Western patients to describe though they have names in Chinese (see p. 12). These sensations may spread around the needle for a variable distance or may travel up or down the limb.

Teh chi

The term teh chi refers collectively to all these phenomena, both those experienced by the acupuncturist and those experienced by the patient. The Chinese attach great significance to teh chi and indeed regard it as essential if a good result is to be achieved; some Western acupuncturists, however, do not regard it as important. My own impression is that it makes a favourable outcome more likely though it is not always essential. In needling TPs I take teh chi to indicate that the needle has entered the right place.

2. General effects

A certain degree of relaxation is so common following acupuncture as to be almost the rule. This may go on to become actual drowsiness; some patients say they feel as if they could go to sleep. This is a pleasant sensation; indeed a minority of patients experience frank euphoria and may compare the feeling to that produced by alcohol or (if they are familiar with it) hashish. These very interesting effects are possibly due to endorphins, although they may come on surprisingly quickly, perhaps within a minute or so of the insertion of the needle, a fact which is difficult to explain in terms of endorphin release. If pronounced, they mark the patient as a *strong reactor*.

Strong reactors

Approximately 2–5 per cent of the population are strong reactors (the exact percentage depends on where one draws the line). Strong reactors may experience localised effects in areas distant from those being treated (for example, needling one foot may cause sensations to be felt in the opposite foot, or in the face). They also experience marked generalised effects such as those just described.

Strong reactors can sometimes be identified before treatment. They are usually young (under 35) and many have a noticeably clear skin and eyes. They may give a history of allergies or adverse reactions to a number of drugs and are often liable to motion sickness. Children should always be regarded as strong reactors.

It is important to recognise strong reactors before treatment if possible, since although they respond exceptionally well to acupuncture they can also easily be made worse by over-enthusiastic treatment. They should be needled at only one or two sites, the needle being inserted for only a short time (perhaps a matter of seconds) and stimulated gently or not at all. Because it is not always possible to recognise strong reactors in advance, *all* new patients should be treated lightly. This not only helps to prevent adverse reactions, but it makes subsequent treatment easier, because if large numbers of points are used on the first occasion and the result is good, the same number of points has to be used next time, whereas if fewer points are used it is easier to see which have been effective.

Some patients who react strongly to the first treatment react much less strongly to the second treatment and hardly at all to the third and subsequent treatments. Such patients are placebo responders and could be called 'pseudo-strong reactors'. True strong reactors, in contrast, continue to experience the same effects every time they are treated, sometimes for years.

3. Complications

Although acupuncture is generally safe, a great many complications have been reported, including some deaths. The following list is not intended to be exhaustive but will give an idea of what to look out for.

Infection

Provided needles are sterilised properly infection should be very rare. The main exception to this concerns the insertion of semi-permanent needles in the ear. These can certainly give rise to local infections and there has been a recent report of a patient who developed a bacterial endocarditis, apparently owing to the insertion of such a needle. Semi-permanent needles should therefore not be used in patients with known abnormalities of their heart valves, but the difficulty here is that valve abnormalities are not always recognised in advance. Some medical acupuncturists are therefore not very happy about using semi-permanent needles at all, especially as they can also give rise to infection of the ear cartilage, which is difficult to treat.

If semi-permanent needles are not used bacterial infection is very unlikely, and the principal risk is transmission of hepatitis. The virus responsible for hepatitis can be carried in a minute amount of blood and there have been cases of hepatitis caused by acupuncture in this country. AIDS is of course another worry, though so far there have been no reports of AIDS being transmitted by acupuncture needles and in fact it seems probable that the amount of blood that an acupuncture needle could carry would be too small to transmit an infective dose of this virus, though this is obviously not a reason for complacency.

The acupuncturist must keep in mind the possibility of infecting himself by means of an accidental needle prick. There is a strong case for considering immunisation against infective hepatitis if one is doing a lot of acupuncture. Dentists are now being officially advised to be immunised against hepatitis, and it seems reasonable for doctors practising acupuncture to take the same precaution. In any case, it is important to be obsessively careful about handling used acupuncture needles, and acupuncture should not be carried out on patients in the recognised high-risk groups for hepatitis and AIDS until they have been shown, by blood tests, not to be carriers.

An important question that arises in connection with preventing infection is whether or not to swab the skin. Although it is customary to wipe the skin with a swab impregnated with alcohol before giving an injection, the evidence that this really achieves a great deal is rather sketchy (Grant, 1986). Certainly it is impossible to sterilise the skin in the sense of removing all the bacteria, but giving it a wipe does diminish the population of bacteria at least temporarily. Whether sufficient bacteria to cause infection would be carried in by an acupuncture needle is doubtful; certainly there are many diabetics who do not wipe the skin before their daily insulin injection and suffer no ill-effects. Nevertheless, there is nothing to be lost by doing so, and just possibly it may prevent the occasional (extremely rare) instance of bacterial infection due to acupuncture. If the skin is cleaned in this way, time should then be allowed for the alcohol to evaporate before the needle is inserted.

These remarks do not apply to patients with known abnormalities of their heart valves or whose immune system is not functioning properly. Such patients are in a different category; their skin should be scrubbed for 2 minutes with chlorhexidine or 1–2% iodine in 70% ethyl alcohol, but it is doubtful if such patients should be treated with acupuncture at all.

Abortion
There are numerous anecdotal reports that acupuncture can induce abortion. While these may be coincidences it is safer to assume that they are not, and pregnancy is therefore a relative (not absolute) contra-indication to acupuncture. If acupuncture is done at this time it should be performed lightly and certain points (Sp6 and the lower back) should be avoided altogether.

Fainting
This is quite common and is no different from the kind of fainting that may occur with any minor surgical procedure. To prevent it, patients who seem at all apprehensive or who are known to faint easily should be treated lying down, at least on the first occasion.

Convulsions
A number of doctors have reported the occurrence of epileptiform seizures during acupuncture. These have usually been in patients with no history of epilepsy. In most cases the patients were sitting at the time and so the likely explanation is that they fainted and the consequent fall in blood supply to the brain caused the convulsion. However, it is also possible that in some cases the convulsion was a direct effect of acupuncture. In this connection it is interesting that one class of opioid receptors in the brain (the delta receptors) is said to be capable of causing epilepsy.

There have been no long-term ill-effects from any of the episodes of convulsions reported so far but they are obviously alarming to the acupuncturist at the time, especially if he is unaware that they may occur.

Sweating and other autonomic effects
Sweating and other autonomic effects are common with acupuncture, but are hardly significant enough to deserve the name of complications. They may be non-specific responses to an alarming situation but they can also occur in patients who are well used to acupuncture and do not mind it; in such cases they are probably specific acupuncture effects.

Haemorrhage
Minor capillary or venous haemorrhage is common and not serious; arterial haemorrhage is very rare, probably because the relatively blunt point of the acupuncture needle tends to push arteries aside rather than penetrate them. Haemorrhage of any kind can be quickly stopped simply by local pressure. If a small haematoma forms, it should be flattened out by massaging it for

a few minutes; this prevents it from being painful later and speeds up its absorption.

Patients should be warned about the possible appearance of a bruise after acupuncture, especially if the needles have been inserted into a visible site such as the face.

Bleeding is said to be more common in patients who are taking aspirin regularly, and it is of course more likely in patients receiving anticoagulants, which are thus at least a relative contra-indication to treatment; the same applies to bleeding disorders such as haemophilia and to drugs that depress the immune system.

Anatomical

The biggest danger in acupuncture is causing damage to internal organs. Almost every organ in the body has been perforated by an acupuncturist at some time or other. The obvious way of preventing this is for the acupuncturist to have a sound knowledge of anatomy. Some of the treatments described in acupuncture books (especially traditional texts) are potentially hazardous and would be avoided by a Western doctor. The commonest serious complication to have occurred in recent years in this country has been pneumothorax, when needles have been inserted into the chest wall. Pneumothorax is not a grave danger for someone in reasonable health but for a patient suffering from emphysema, who may have little spare lung capacity, it can prove fatal. Pneumothorax may not come on until some hours after acupuncture and may not be immediately detectable even on a radiograph.

Needle fracture

Needles may break off in the tissues. To avoid this, discard needles that are bent or corroded. Applying moxa to the handle (not recommended anyway) can cause weakening.

Needles can become hooked at the tip, especially after periosteal stimulation; the hook can often be felt, rather than seen, if the needle is wiped on the sterile swab before insertion. Such needles cause undesirable pain and trauma and should be discarded.

Contra-indications: a summary
The foregoing list may seem rather intimidating but it has to be recognised that any medical procedure carries some risks; only useless treatments are entirely safe. In practice, acupuncture is remarkably free from serious dangers, provided it is competently carried out.

The following summary lists the main contra-indications to acupuncture (A=absolute, R=relative).

   (a) Patients known or suspected to be carriers of hepatitis or AIDS (A).
   (b) Patients who are afraid or unwilling to have acupuncture (R).
   (c) Pregnancy, especially in the first trimester (R).
   (d) Bleeding disorders (R).
   (e) Skin infections (R).
   (f) Valvular heart disease (R: A if insertion of semi-permanent needles is contemplated).
   (g) Disorders of the immune system (R).

EFFECT OF ACUPUNCTURE ON SYMPTOMS

Improvement, if it occurs, may be immediate or may take some hours or days to appear. Improvements that take a little time to appear sometimes seem to last longer than those that come on immediately. The duration of any improvement is likewise uncertain; improvement occurring after the first one or two treatments is often short-lived but with subsequent treatments it may last longer.

Aggravations (that is, worsening of existing symptoms) are quite common. They may indicate that treatment has been too vigorous, but some patients regularly experience aggravations after every treatment and come to expect them. Aggravations seldom last more than 48 hours, though exceptionally they may continue for a week or more. They are usually though not invariably followed by an improvement. Patients should be warned about their possible occurrence.

Non-responders
About 30 per cent of the population appear to be incapable of

responding to acupuncture. This becomes evident after they have been treated a few times without success but it can be suspected if there is no apparent response at the time of needling to even quite strong stimulation. It is not clear why certain patients should show this lack of response, but it is important to realise that it occurs.

FREQUENCY OF TREATMENT

There can be no general rule about this. Acute disease may need frequent treatment, but chronic disease is usually treated less frequently (though some patients may benefit from daily treatment for a time). Since improvement can take up to a week to appear it is seldom desirable to treat chronic disease more often than once a week.

There can also be no general rule about how many treatments are required. A commonly seen pattern of response is that the first treatment produces a transient and partial improvement; the second treatment produces a greater and more sustained improvement, and this continues up to perhaps the fourth or sixth treatment, after which a 'plateau' of improvement is reached. However, the effects of any individual treatment are hard to predict; one may achieve a lot, while the next seems to do little or nothing.

As a rule it is not worth treating any given patient more than three times if there is no effect at all. It is, however, important to question the patient closely to make sure that there really has been no response, because some people do not realise that a brief improvement after the first treatment, lasting perhaps only 24 or 48 hours, is significant, and may say that the acupuncture did nothing.

In some circumstances it may be worth trying acupuncture more than three times in the absence of a response; for example, if the patient is very insistent, if there is no other treatment available, if the problem is one that *ought* to respond to acupuncture, or in certain disorders (such as sciatica) which sometimes respond slowly. It requires experience to know in which cases it may be justifiable to persist for some time in the absence of a clear improvement.

It is important to understand that in many cases acupuncture does not *cure* disease (chronic disease, anyway); rather, it relieves the symptoms for a variable length of time. Many patients will therefore require 'boosters' at intervals ranging from a few weeks to several months. If the remission period is still too short even after a number of treatments it must be concluded that acupuncture has failed. There is no fixed length of time that constitutes the minimum acceptable duration of a remission, but in my own practice I tend to regard six weeks as the cut-off point. However, this is not an absolute rule, and it has to be recognised that there are some patients for whom rather shorter periods of improvement may still be worth while.

When symptoms keep coming back after an initial treatment one needs to identify things that may be perpetuating them. These may include environmental, psychological and postural factors, which should be removed or corrected if possible. If such factors cannot be identified or cannot be altered, it may sometimes be a solution to teach patients to carry out self-acupuncture. Alternatively, transcutaneous electrical nerve stimulation (TENS) (see Chapter 9) may help.

Claims are sometimes made that acupuncture can 'reverse pathology'; that is, alter disease processes and so bring about a true 'cure'. Unfortunately there is little good evidence for this. It seems reasonable to assume that acupuncture can restore normal function (by inactivating TPs or in other ways) and that this can sometimes halt disease at an early stage. It seems much less likely that it can alter established pathology, but the distinction is not always clear cut. For example, acupuncture can sometimes relieve the pain of duodenal ulcer, but there is no good evidence that it can actually heal ulcers. Yet some animal experiments do seem to have shown that it can alter the pattern of blood flow in the duodenum, so just conceivably it could heal ulcers. In the absence of proper clinical trials it is impossible to know, but it seems safer to assume that it cannot. This rather cautious assumption at least prevents one from being lulled into a false sense of security; the fact that a symptom is relieved by acupuncture does not necessarily mean that there is no serious underlying disease. (I have already mentioned (p. 37) that acupuncture can relieve the headache due to brain tumour.)

As a working hypothesis, I assume that acupuncture can help to bring about recovery that could in principle occur by the unaided efforts of nature, but nothing more. This is not so gloomy as it may sound. The degree of pain or disability that a patient suffers frequently (in fact, usually) bears little or no relationship to the changes revealed by radiographic and other investigations, so that even though acupuncture is largely a symptomatic treatment this is not to say it is valueless.

INTRODUCING ACUPUNCTURE TO NEW PATIENTS

Unless a patient has come with the specific intention of receiving acupuncture, the doctor will have to suggest it. I think it is usually best to do this indirectly, saying something like: 'I think I might be able to help you if you don't mind my putting in one or two plain needles.' This usually then leads into a discussion of acupuncture. In any case, it is important to spend some time explaining the procedure for every new patient, to give her as clear an idea as possible what to expect. In particular, the common question 'Does it hurt?' should be answered truthfully. Some kinds of treatment hurt hardly at all, while others hurt a fair amount. In the case of TP needling I rely on the patient to tell me when the needle is in the right place, so this is inevitably somewhat painful. All this has to be explained. As a standard of comparison, I usually say that acupuncture hurts less than the average visit to the dentist and rather less than the average injection.

In his book on acupuncture, Dr Alexander Macdonald (1984) suggests that the doctor should demonstrate the technique on himself. Although I agree that any acupuncturist worth his salt should be able to do this, I have found that such demonstrations are seldom reassuring to apprehensive patients; quite the reverse, in fact. If verbal explanations do not reassure a patient I normally would not carry out acupuncture on her, at least on that occasion. It is better to send her away and ask her to think it over and perhaps discuss the idea with a relative.

For patients who are afraid of acupuncture there are some alternatives that can be tried. Sometimes firm pressure on a TP for a few minutes will inactivate it, at least temporarily. Travell's and Simon's 'stretch and spray' technique can be used, or some form of TENS can be tried.

In general, selecting the right patients to treat is as important as selecting the right points to needle, possibly more so.

REFERENCES

Grant, A. J. (1986). Skin swabbing. *Acupuncture in Medicine*, **3**, 15.

Macdonald, A. (1984). *Acupuncture: From Ancient Art to Modern Medicine*, p. 4. George Allen and Unwin, London.

Chapter Five
GENERAL PRINCIPLES

Among the questions often asked about acupuncture are:
1. What disorders are suitable for treatment?
2. Where should the needles be placed?
3. How deep should the needles be inserted?
The full answers to these questions can only come with experience, but it is possible to lay down a few guidelines.

WHAT DISORDERS ARE SUITABLE FOR TREATMENT?

Quite often in acupuncture one is dealing not so much with a pathological diagnosis (for example, osteoarthrosis) as with a symptom or symptom complex (pain in the neck, pain in the shoulder, and so on). This does not of course mean that one should not try to reach a pathological diagnosis if possible, but rather that in many cases a pathological diagnosis is not attainable or is irrelevant. This applies particularly in the case of radiological changes in the spine. These changes, which may be described to the patient as 'arthritis' or, alternatively, 'wear and tear', are very common by middle age and almost universal by 65. On the other hand, by no means everyone in these age ranges experiences symptoms either continuously or at all, and in fact there is very little correspondence between the radiological appearances and symptoms. Of course, in any individual case the radiological changes *may* explain the symptoms but it should not be assumed uncritically that they do so, nor should it be concluded that because there are severe changes the chances of improvement with acupuncture are nil. The main reason for ordering radiographs in back pain is not to try to explain the symptoms as due to 'arthritis' but to exclude other, rarer, causes for back pain.

Acupuncture can certainly be used when there is objective evidence, such as radiological changes, for anatomical and pathological abnormalities, but it can also be very helpful when, as often happens, the most elaborate investigations fail to show anything amiss. In such cases the patient is often labelled as suffering from a 'functional' disorder, which is usually a code word meaning that the symptoms are 'psychological'. While this is undoubtedly often the case, there are also many patients whose symptoms are 'functional' in a different, more useful, sense; that is, they are due to disordered *function*, which is frequently associated with TPs.

For descriptive purposes it is convenient to divide the disorders suitable for treatment by acupuncture into two broad groups: musculoskeletal disorders and other treatable disorders. The distinction is not rigid and TPs play an important part in many of the 'other' disorders, but it simplifies the discussion.

For musculoskeletal disorders acupuncture is often the treatment of choice provided patients are willing to have it. It is probably safer than the anti-inflammatory drugs commonly used in such cases and is often more effective. As regards 'other' disorders there are wide variations. These disorders can be roughly classified into three groups:

Group A: Disorders or symptoms that usually respond to acupuncture (50–70 per cent).

Group B: Disorders that respond moderately well (20–50 per cent).

Group C: Disorders that seldom or never respond (less than 10 per cent).

When I talk to new patients who have not specifically asked for acupuncture I usually suggest it for Group A. For Group B I am more cautious and only suggest it if I think, for one reason or another, that they are fairly likely to respond. For Group C I would normally not use acupuncture though I might do so if the patient was very insistent (which makes it more likely that acupuncture will work), if no other available treatment seemed to offer a chance of success, or if the patient was likely to be a strong reactor. (Being a strong reactor moves a patient up by at least one category.)

Musculoskeletal disorders are for the most part equivalent to Group A disorders in terms of their response to treatment.

WHERE SHOULD THE NEEDLES BE PLACED?

This is of course the central question in acupuncture, or at least it is likely to seem so to the beginner. Unfortunately it has to be said that there are almost as many opinions about needle placement as there are practitioners of acupuncture. However, the main possibilities are as follows.

(a) *Traditional*: The points are chosen in accordance with the traditional Chinese theories of channels, yin-yang, and so on.

(b) *Neoclassical*: The points are chosen in accordance with a modern re-interpretation of the traditional ideas. Electrical instruments may or may not be used in these methods, and there may be little resemblance to the ancient system; however, concepts of 'energy balancing' are usually retained.

(c) *Cook book* (see below): This is a very simplified version of the traditional system, lacking any theoretical foundation but relying on the concepts of points and channels.

(d) *Painful area/segmental*: The sites to be needled are selected on the basis of modern knowledge of the spinal segments, so that the needles are inserted in the relevant dermatome. In its simplest form, this method consists simply in needling the painful area itself.

(e) *Trigger point*: TPs are used.

(f) *Single point*: Occasionally just one point is used for all patients (for example, G41 to treat tension headaches). Such drastic simplification has characterised some research studies but few doctors practising routine acupuncture take their scepticism about the existence of acupuncture points as far as this.

My own approach is eclectic and makes use of most of the above possibilities on occasion; however, it is mainly based on (d) and (e) though with the addition of certain traditional acupuncture points. For the most part I consider these as sites at which it is possible to produce a profound *generalised* effect, though as indicated in Chapter 2 I keep open the possibility that at least some of the traditional points may have specific effects. I find that, in common with many other doctors practising acupuncture, my ideas about this fascinating subject are in a state of constant flux and, I hope, development; which is as it should be.

The 'cook-book' approach
Most beginners in acupuncture start by using a 'cook book'. This is a book that lists the acupuncture points to use in various disorders. The method has severe limitations, which stem from its failure to provide any kind of insight into what is going on.

To pursue the cooking metaphor a little, the acupuncturist who relies on a 'cook book' is like a cook who slavishly follows her recipes. Excusable in a beginner, this procedure cannot yield interesting results for very long. No good cook adheres rigidly to the ingredients and quantities laid down in the recipes; instead, as her experience increases she begins to acquire insight into the underlying principles of cooking and so can make her own adaptations of the recipes to suit her own tastes and those of her family or the contents of her larder. In the end she may well come to make up her own recipes in increasing independence of all recipe books.

Like the good cook, the acupuncturist should aim at becoming independent. In fact, at this point the metaphor breaks down, for while even experienced cooks may still use recipe books on occasion and indeed are likely to possess a large number of them, almost the only real use of acupuncture cook books is to supply confidence for the beginner, and the sooner they are left behind the better.

If you look at an acupuncture cook book you will find that the choice of points is largely governed by two main principles. Some of the points are situated in the neighbourhood of the affected area, while others are remote from it on channels that run near it. Thus facial pain, for example, might be treated by a combination of Bladder, Gall bladder and Stomach points on the face plus Bladder or Gall bladder points on the feet. If one thinks about this in non-traditional terms, one realises that the local points can be regarded as TPs, while the distant points may also be TPs but in addition are chosen for reasons connected with channel theory.

For the modern acupuncturist, much of the art consists in the detection and treatment of TPs, which may well also be classical acupuncture points; however, the important thing is that they are TPs, and local tenderness is the criterion of choice rather than correspondence to a site described in a classical text. The vast majority of these TPs are situated in or fairly near the affected area, and in my experience it is seldom an advantage to needle very distant acupuncture points, at least in the treatment of painful disorders.

From what I have just said it can be seen that the modern acupuncturist uses a combination of points, of which some are classical acupuncture points and some are not. This may seem rather untidy but it works in practice.

Even though the modern acupuncturist may be sceptical about the objective existence of some or all acupuncture points, a working knowledge of the location of at least the more important points is needed, for two reasons. First, when attending acupuncture meetings or reading books or papers on acupuncture, one will encounter the traditional terminology; a knowledge of the main acupuncture points is thus required for literacy in the subject. Second, in treating patients it is essential to keep a record of what one has done, and the traditional terminology provides a convenient shorthand for the purpose.

In practice, I tend to use a mixture of traditional acupuncture and modern anatomical terms to list the points I have treated. If there is a traditional point at or close to the site I have needled I write it down, otherwise I use a description based on Western anatomical terms. I also record the side needled (R or L or both) together with any other relevant information, such as the duration of needling and the effects, if any. Thus an initial treatment might be recorded as follows:

Liv3×2 (2 min): general reaction ++ (euphoria)
or:
Vastus medialis TP (R): painful ++
Gluteus medius TP (R): painful ++

Yet another way of recording one's results is to mark them on a drawing of the body. Rubber stamps are available for this purpose. Whatever method one adopts, it should be clear to oneself on re-reading the notes as well as to anyone else who may have to treat the patient in the future.

Although the classic texts list hundreds of acupuncture points, in practice far fewer were commonly used. The modern acupuncturist may conveniently cut down the list very considerably, to include only those points which are used frequently and whose locations should therefore be known by heart. No doubt everyone would have a slightly different list of such points, but here, for what it is worth, is my own 'top ten': (See pages 96–8 for charts illustrating their location.)
Liv 3
Sp6
S36
B57
B23
GV15
G20
G21
CV17
LI 4

HOW DEEP SHOULD THE NEEDLES BE INSERTED?

The obvious, if unhelpful, answer to this question is, 'as deep as necessary'. It is all a question of what one is trying to achieve. In all cases the needle should go right through the skin, since intradermal acupuncture is very painful. Much modern acupuncture is concerned with TPs, and in my experience it is essential to needle the TP as accurately as possible. Most TPs are in muscle and it is therefore essential to put the point of the needle into the muscle concerned. Sometimes the TP is fairly superficial, in which case it can be reached with a 30mm needle, but sometimes it is deep (for example, in the back or the buttocks), in which case a 50mm needle will be required. (See Chapter 6 for a more detailed discussion of the technique of needling TPs.)

An alternative approach is not to needle the TP directly but instead to insert several needles quite superficially (into but not beyond the subcutaneous tissue) at half-inch intervals over the TP. The needles are left in longer with this technique than with direct needling. Its advantage is that it is almost painless; the disadvantage, for me at least, is that I find it usually less effective. For a few patients, however, it is actually more effective than the standard techique, so it is a useful addition to the acupuncturist's repertoire.

Needling at classic acupuncture points which are not TPs is normally into muscle; the depth in these cases is usually about half an inch (1.25cm).

Periosteal acupuncture, as the name implies, consists in needling the periosteum. This technique, which was first described by Dr Felix Mann, is useful in the treatment of certain musculoskeletal disorders (see Chapter 6). The needle is inserted to whatever depth is required to reach the periosteum (or, in some cases, ligaments or other deep structures); 50mm needles may be required for this.

Chapter Six
THE TREATMENT OF
MUSCULOSKELETAL DISORDERS

GENERAL CONSIDERATIONS

In acupuncture one is to some extent working outside the usual
medical categories and is more concerned with symptom
patterns than with formal pathological diagnosis. Even so, it
must not be forgotten that acupuncture is part of medicine and
the underlying disease process should always be kept in mind in
so far as it is known. What appears to be a straightforward
musculoskeletal problem may really be a manifestation of a
serious underlying disorder such as an infection or cancer. *In
this chapter and in Chapter 7 it is assumed that all the
investigations that may be indicated have been carried out. It
would be outside the scope of this book to discuss all the
diagnostic possibilities for each of the symptom complexes I have
included, and I have concentrated on the acupuncture aspects;
but the importance of accurate diagnosis cannot be over-
emphasised.*

The type of acupuncture treatment chosen, and even the
decision to use acupuncture at all, is of course influenced by the
pathological diagnosis. On the whole, acupuncture is most
useful in disorders of function, though it can also be helpful
when there is obvious pathology. In such cases it does not alter
the damage in the tissues but it can modify the secondary effects
of damage such as pain and stiffness.

In inflammatory disorders such as rheumatoid arthritis it

certainly is not curative, and I do not myself think it has much part to play in the treatment of widespread rheumatoid arthritis. However, it can be very helpful if the disease is predominantly affecting only one or two joints. But needles should not be inserted in the vicinity of acutely swollen hot joints.

Much the commonest type of musculoskeletal disorder that the acupuncturist encounters is pain arising from the spine. Many words have been written about this distressingly common affliction and this in itself is a sure sign that the problem is poorly understood. I certainly do not intend to enter the controversy here; nevertheless it is necessary to have some kind of scheme in mind as one approaches one's patient, needle in hand.

A common and natural question from the patient is, 'Do I have arthritis?' This can be difficult to answer. A radiograph of the spine in a middle-aged man or woman is very likely to show various abnormalities such as loss of the normal disc spaces and other distortions of the normal architecture. These changes are referred to collectively as spondylosis, and many authorities, though not all, regard them as a fully adequate cause of symptoms such as pain in the neck or back, pain down the arms or legs, tingling or numbness in the limbs, and so on. The usual explanation given is that the spinal nerves are being compressed as they come between the vertebrae and that this compression is responsible for all the symptoms.

However, many people who have no symptoms at all will have abnormal radiographs, and conversely many people with symptoms will have normal radiographs, so the matter is not as simple as it first appears. There is no doubt that nerve compression does occur as a result of spinal degeneration, but what is at issue is whether this is the only, or even the commonest, cause of symptoms. The question is important, because if one believes that the symptoms are the inevitable result of changes in the spine that come with ageing, it follows that the patient must expect to get gradually worse, with little hope of relief except from pain-relieving drugs, with their potentially dangerous side-effects.

In fact, however, one knows that neck and back pain does not necessarily get worse as time goes by; in fact, it may last from weeks to months but shows a tendency to get better by itself. Some authors, and in particular Travell and Simons, explain this, to my mind convincingly, by an alternative theory.

While admitting that nerve entrapment in the spinal column does occur, they believe that a more frequent cause of pain is referral from trigger points (TPs) in the muscles and other tissues. This idea is supported by the fact that treatment aimed at eliminating the TPs does, in many cases, relieve the patient's symptoms.

A useful classification of pain of spinal origin has been put forward by J. P. O'Brien (1984); I shall use it here, in a slightly modified form.

Type A pain is dull, deep, and aching in quality and is poorly localised. It may be felt in the back or may radiate to distant areas as *referred pain*. There may also be altered patterns of sensation in these areas. The distribution of this pain is fairly constant but it does not correspond to the known areas of supply of nerves or nerve roots. This 'sclerotome pain' may radiate to the eye, chest wall, elbow, groin, lower abdomen, or foot, and not surprisingly can give rise to problems in diagnosis. It may also be referred to the sacro-iliac joint, which sometimes leads to mistaken diagnosis of sacro-iliac strain. The sacro-iliac joint can in fact be a source of pain, but this is typically felt over the ischial tuberosity and down the thigh to the knee.

Type A pain is the kind most typically associated with TPs.

Type B pain arises from the superficial tissues (skin, fascia, superficial ligaments and muscles, tips of spinous processes). It is felt at the site of trouble and is accurately localised.

Type C pain is due to involvement of the spinal nerves or sympathetic trunk. Stimulation of a spinal nerve causes sharp 'electric' superficial pain in a dermatome distribution. (The pain which results from striking the ulnar nerve – the 'funny bone' – is of this kind.) There may be paralysis, paraesthesiae, or anaesthesia, and muscular weakness or loss of reflexes.

Although Type C pain is described as having a dermatome distribution, it has to be remembered that the accuracy of the dermatome charts is uncertain and indeed the dermatomes are not entirely fixed entities but can change in area and distribution in the same individual.

Involvement of the sympathetic nerves may cause vascular changes or pain, though the exact pain patterns are not known precisely.

From this brief discussion it will be clear that the patterns of pain and altered sensation that can occur in spinal disorders are complex and often it is not possible to be certain about what is the cause of the symptoms experienced by any given patient. So far as acupuncture is concerned, however, it is possible to draw certain conclusions. Acupuncture can be useful in the treatment of Type A and Type B pain, but has little effect in Type C pain.

From the acupuncture point of view, the presence or absence of TPs is a most important additional consideration in any case of spinal pain; TPs form a kind of counterpoint to the main theme of musculoskeletal pain. In general, acupuncture is more likely to be successful in patients who have TPs, although the chances of success are not neglible in their absence.

EXAMINING THE PATIENT

In treating musculoskeletal disorders with acupuncture, the first essential is to assess the patient's appearance, posture and mobility. Many clues can be obtained by the ease, or difficulty, with which she walks, undresses and lies down and turns over on the couch.

Next, a search is made for TPs. It is important to place the muscle or muscles to be examined in a position of slight tension. Various methods of looking for TPs have been described, including the use of mechanical and electrical probes, but in most cases the most useful tool is the examiner's finger. The area is carefully searched, using light pressure at first and then progressively heavier pressure. In this way both the degree of sensitivity of any TPs found as well as their approximate depth can be estimated.

TPs can be felt in many cases, but the technique has to be learned by practical demonstration. The tips, rather than the pads, of the fingers are used, and are drawn *transversely* across the muscle fibres; Travell and Simons (1984a) compare the action to that of feeling corduroy. If TPs are in muscle they often take the form of rather ill-defined bands of taut muscle, while in the subcutaneous tissues they may present as nodules. The most characteristic feature of TPs, however, is that they are tender to pressure.

Pressing a TP gives rise to pain which may be anything from slight to agonising. The pain is felt at the site of pressure and sometimes may also cause pain to radiate to areas of referred pain. In exceptional cases pressure on a TP will reproduce the patient's symptoms exactly or will relieve them; when this occurs the chances of effecting an improvement with acupuncture are excellent.

One difficulty is to distinguish between TPs and sites of referred pain. This is not always easy but it is important, since needling sites of referred pain is seldom beneficial and indeed may worsen the patient's symptoms. Travell and Simons (1984b) make a useful distinction between *satellite TPs*, in the zone of referred pain, and *secondary TPs*, in synergist or antagonist muscles. The number of TPs varies considerably, from one or two to dozens. If they are very numerous, improvement may be difficult to achieve.

Other TP effects in addition to pain may occur. For example, pressure on a TP can cause muscular twitching; this can often be demonstrated in the forearm muscles (extensor digitorum) if these are plucked like a guitar string, when the middle finger may jerk upwards; this is said to be a muscle response rather than a spinal reflex since it still occurs if the nerve supply to the muscle is blocked with an injection of local anaesthetic. Autonomic effects can also occur when TPs are stimulated.

An important clinical sign is the 'jump sign': pressure on a very active TP causes the patient to flinch or 'jump' and sometimes exclaim in pain.

THE TREATMENT OF SPECIFIC REGIONS

The neck region

Examination and treatment are most conveniently carried out with the patient sitting, the acupuncturist standing behind her; but the caution about treating patients sitting should be kept in mind. If there is any question of the patient's fainting, she can be placed sitting on the couch with her back towards the acupuncturist; in this position she can quickly be laid flat if necessary.

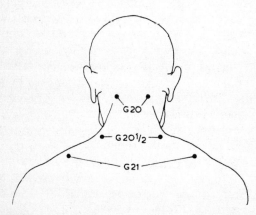

Fig. 6/1 Posterior view of the head and neck showing points G20, G20½, G21

The commonest sites for TPs are G21, G20, and a point midway between the two at the angle between neck and shoulders; this is not a recognised acupuncture point but it may be conveniently labelled G20½. In anatomical terms, G21 is situated in the upper trapezius, G20½ in the levator scapulae, and G20 in the posterior cervical muscles (Fig. 6/1). All these are usually treated routinely for neck pain; both sides are treated though more attention is given to the painful side.

Other muscles that may be involved include rhomboideus major and minor, supraspinatus and infraspinatus; there is quite often another TP in the lower trapezius, either between the scapulae or below the lower angle of the scapula.

Particular care should be taken when needling G21 because of the proximity of the lung, which rises above the first rib and may be quite close to the surface in thin people. To avoid piercing the pleura the needle should not be inserted at right angles to the skin but should be passed more or less parallel to the skin and no deeper than 30mm.

In addition to these points there may be TPs in the neck muscles overlying the cervical vertebrae. These can be detected by compressing the muscles against the bone and can be treated by needling. In his book *The Treatment of Disease by Acupuncture*, Mann (1980) describes the technique of needling the transverse processes of the cervical vertebrae, which he finds more effective than needling muscles in this region. I have not found so much difference myself and I prefer to avoid needling these vertebrae because of the theoretical risk of injuring the vertebral artery.

Pain from these TPs can be referred to various sites, including the back of the head, the forehead and the eyes, and also the shoulders and arms. It follows that the neck should always be examined, and usually treated, when there is pain in these distant areas.

Shoulder pain

Pain in the shoulder is a problem that is often brought to the acupuncturist. It may be extrinsic (referred) or intrinsic. There are many causes of extrinsic shoulder pain, including neck disorders, but also others such as disease of the gall bladder or heart and various tumours. Intrinsic shoulder pain can be due to arthritis and various less common causes; however, it is sobering to record that Dr Virginia Camp (1986), a rheumatologist who uses acupuncture, found in the course of five years 12 patients with a diagnosis of frozen shoulder in whom the pain was actually a manifestation of a serious disorder; 8 of them had cancer of various kinds and another had leukaemia. These cases emphasise the importance of making a proper pathological diagnosis whenever possible.

The majority of the patients who come to the doctor practising acupuncture, however, will have a frozen shoulder. This is a little-understood disorder; a recent review by Bunker (1985) came to the conclusion that there is at present no agreement about either its cause or the best way to treat it.

A frozen shoulder may come on gradually or suddenly. The amount of pain varies but it can be very severe, requiring morphine or similar strong drugs to relieve it. There is always some loss of movement but this too is variable; in severe cases movement at the shoulder is totally lost, though the patient can still use the arm to some extent by moving the scapula.

In many patients, but by no means all, the disease gradually improves spontaneously and recovery is complete within about a year. The pain goes first and movement returns more slowly; many patients do not recover full movement although they may not be aware of this. Even after five years, a certain number of patients will still have symptoms.

Once recovery has occurred the disease does not normally recur, although sometimes the opposite shoulder is affected later.

Two main types of frozen shoulder are usually described. One form is said to be due to adhesive capsulitis. In this variety, both active and passive movements are restricted in all planes. The other form is due to lesions of the rotator cuff or other muscles and tendons around the joint. This type gives rise to pain on active and resisted movement in particular planes. Cyriax (1982a) has described detailed methods of examining the shoulder in order to separate out the various structures that may be at fault, and his books make the matter seem quite clear and logical. In practice, unfortunately, things are often not so simple, and other factors seem to be at work.

The situation is not any better when we come to treatment. A wide range of treatments is advocated by different authors, including rest, exercises, physiotherapy, corticosteroid injections, anti-inflammatory drugs, manipulation under anaesthesia, as well as acupuncture. It is not clear that any one of these is better than the rest; all seem to help on occasion, but clinical trials seem to suggest that in most cases the disease follows its own course regardless of treatment. It is interesting that one study which compared the effects of acupuncture, physiotherapy, injection plus oral anti-inflammatory drugs and placebo, found no differences among any of the treatments, all of which seemed to produce good results (Berry et al, 1980).

So far as acupuncture is concerned, my impression is that it can help some patients considerably and is certainly worth a try provided the symptoms are not too severe, in which case the patient requires strong analgesics. Acupuncture seems to relieve mild to moderate pain quite well, though often it does so for only rather short periods; it therefore needs to be repeated fairly frequently, and I am not convinced that it shortens the period of disability from what it would otherwise be.

To treat a painful shoulder with acupuncture, one first makes a careful examination for TPs. The common sites of TPs, in addition to those already mentioned, are the coracoid process and the groove in front of the humerus in which the tendon of the long head of the biceps lies. Both can be needled deeply (that is, periosteal needling). In some cases the problem seems to lie in the supraspinatus tendon, in which case the needle should be passed into the tendon beneath the acromion.

I do not often use remote points for treatment of this kind of pain, but it is sometimes helpful to treat SI 3 and LI 4 in the hand.

The upper limbs

The elbow
Pain in the elbow is most commonly located at the lateral epicondyle of the humerus (so-called tennis elbow). In these cases there is usually exquisite tenderness over the bony prominence and the most logical treatment would seem to be to needle this periosteally. Although this is sometimes very effective it quite often fails. Possibly this is because one has failed to locate the TP accurately enough, but in many cases it may be because the painful spot is actually a site of referred

pain, the real TP being elsewhere. It is important to make a careful examination of the patient's neck and also of her extensor forearm muscles, where TPs may be found. The lower part of the brachioradialis should also be checked.

Similar considerations apply to the less common golfer's elbow (pain at the medial epicondyle of the humerus).

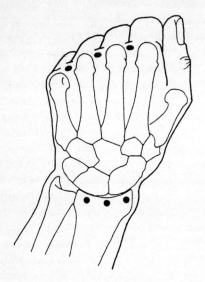

Fig. 6/2 The hand and wrist showing sites for needling

The wrist and hand

Pain in the wrist often seems to respond to periosteal needling at three or four non-specific sites at the lower end of the radius (Fig. 6/2). As always, however, it is important to look carefully for TPs, especially in the shoulders and forearm muscles. An interesting pain pattern sometimes encountered is the finding of an acutely tender point in the wrist, which may be quite localised over one or another carpal bone. It would be natural to expect this to be due to, say, osteoarthritis, but patients with this symptom may also have active TPs in the extensor muscles of the forearm, and needling these can dramatically relieve the tenderness at the wrist. Some cases of 'tenosynovitis' at the wrist are also due to TPs in these muscles.

Case studies:
1. A middle-aged man had been subject to recurrent episodes of pain in the right wrist, brought on by unaccustomed use of the hand (for example, prolonged typing) and also by sleeping with the hand in an awkward position. During the painful episodes a point in the wrist, situated over the capitate bone, would become acutely tender to pressure. Local massage to this point made no difference; however, examination of his right forearm showed active TPs in the extensor muscles (extensor digitorum). 'Plucking' the affected muscles produced a twitch in the relevant fingers and the TPs were markedly tender to pressure. Accurate needling of these TPs gave rise to the characteristic teh chi (p. 49) sensations and abolished the pain at the wrist. The pain recurred after about 10 days but a further treatment produced lasting relief.

2. A middle-aged man was found to have rheumatoid arthritis, the blood tests being positive for this disease. Rather unusually, he also had very large axillary lymph nodes; a biopsy was taken from these and they were reported as being due to rheumatoid arthritis. The only joint to be seriously involved by the disease was his left wrist, which was moderately warm and swollen, with limitation of its movements. He was treated by periosteal acupuncture to the lower end of the radius. Each treatment gave about three months' relief of pain, and gradually, over a three-year period, the swelling of the wrist improved and its mobility increased. The enlarged axillary lymph nodes also shrank to normal.

No doubt the progressive improvement in this patient's condition was due to natural remission, but acupuncture kept him largely pain free during the time of disease activity with none of the side-effects that might have occurred from anti-inflammatory drugs.

3. A worker in an engineering works found that he was

suffering from weakness in his hands, which sometimes caused him to be unable to sustain the weight of heavy loads. He was a powerful man who hitherto had had no such difficulties. Investigations did not show any cause for his weakness, but moderately active TPs were present in the flexor muscles of his forearms. Needling these produced a considerable improvement which lasted for a year, when the symptoms recurred but were relieved by a further course of treatment.

Pain in the hands

Any TPs in the neck, shoulders, or forearms should be treated in the usual way, but in addition it can be helpful to needle the hands themselves. The most useful points are generally LI 4 and the spaces between the knuckles, the needle being passed in at these points in a direction parallel with the metacarpal bones; that is, into the interossei. Alternatively, the needle may be inserted between the metacarpals from the dorsum of the hand; the Chinese describe some 'extra-meridian' points in this situation.

Travell and Simons (1983a) believe that TPs in the interossei may lead to the development of Heberden's nodes. Although these nodules which develop on the sides of the terminal phalanges are usually regarded as manifestations of osteoarthritis, their cause is not understood. They begin as soft tissue swellings, at which time they are tender, but later they become hard but pain free. An interesting feature is that they require an intact nerve supply to develop. They are much commoner in women than in men, and tend to develop around the time of the menopause. Travell and Simons claim that the nodes may disappear completely if the TPs in the interossei are treated.

Pain localised to the base of the thumb is a common clinical problem. This is commonly, but probably often wrongly, ascribed to osteoarthritis of the metacarpophalangeal joint. In fact it is frequently referred from TPs in the forearm extensors or the lower part of the brachioradialis.

The thoracic region

On the whole the thoracic region is more difficult to treat by acupuncture than either the cervical or the lumbar regions. Pain in the thoracic spine is often particularly troublesome. For anatomical reasons it is undesirable to stimulate the periosteum of the thoracic vertebrae, except for the vertebral spines, and this limits the kinds of treatment that can be used. Needling the paraspinal muscles in the thoracic region is possible but is not always very effective. There is however a remote point that can be helpful in such cases; this is SI 3, at the ulnar border of the hand. Although I do not generally find remote points very useful in musculoskeletal problems this is an exception, and SI 3 is worth trying in such cases; it can be needled on one or both sides. The exact location of the point may not be important and possibly anywhere on the hand would do equally well.

Unexplained pain in the chest wall is quite a common problem. Investigations reveal nothing amiss but the pain persists and indeed may last for years. This is a gratifying disorder to treat with acupuncture. Sometimes a TP will be found at a distance from the painful area, perhaps in the spinal region, but usually the treatment consists simply in needling the painful area itself. Often it is enough to put in two or three needles quite superficially, but sometimes it is better to stimulate the periosteum of the rib or ribs in the affected area. In a thin patient this can be done easily and safely by placing a finger on each side of the rib and passing the needle in perpendicularly between them, but if the rib is covered too thickly by fat or muscle, periosteal stimulation should not be attempted for fear of inducing a pneumothorax.

Abdomen

TPs may develop in the abdominal wall just as in the thoracic region and can be treated similarly, but in this area needling must be fairly superficial; several needles should be inserted at intervals of 1 to 2cm into the subcutaneous tissue, but no deeper. One important kind of abdominal pain that can sometimes be helped with acupuncture is pain in the site of surgical scars. This may be associated with acutely tender TPs in the scar itself, in which case they should be needled, but if not it may be helpful simply to insert needles quite superficially around the scar. Sometimes just one treatment of this kind will relieve pain for months or even indefinitely. If acupuncture does not help in such a case one should think about TENS (see Chapter 9).

Low back pain and sciatica

Low back pain is one of the commonest painful disorders that the human organism is subject to. Almost every article on the subject begins with a statement about the frequency of the problem and the number of days of work that are lost annually. It is also one of the least understood diseases; theories abound, but there is no agreement about either its cause or its treatment. It is hardly surprising, therefore, that, together with neck pain, low back pain is one of the main disorders treated by acupuncturists.

There is no space here to go into all the possible causes of low back pain, but it is important to remember that this is, perhaps more than any other, a disorder in which it is essential to keep in mind the wide range of such possibilities. Pain in the back can be due to many local causes including inflammation and malignancy, and it can also be referred to the back from various internal organs. A complaint of low back pain must therefore always be set in the context of a general medical examination, and the minimum investigations required are a full blood count and measurement of the sedimentation rate, together with radiological examination. The purpose of the latter is not so much to reveal degenerative changes such as disc narrowing, which is very common and bears little relation to the presence or severity of symptoms, as to exclude serious pathology such as malignancy or inflammatory arthritis.

Acute low back pain is likely to afflict at least half the adult population at some time during their lives. Sometimes the onset is abrupt and occurs when the patient bends over; his back 'locks' and he cannot straighten up. More often, however, it begins as an ache – lumbago – in the lower back, associated with a variable degree of muscle spasm, which may be severe enough to prevent the patient from tying his shoelaces. This pain persists for some days or weeks, and then usually gets better gradually, with or witout treatment. About 70 per cent of patients recover within three weeks and 90 per cent recover within eight weeks; after six months only 2 or 3 per cent will still have symptoms and thus have entered the chronic stage.

An acute attack of low back pain may or may not be associated with sciatica. This term indicates symptoms of nerve root compression in the leg. Strictly speaking it should be applied only to symptoms connected with the sciatic nerve, but in fact it is often applied to any nerve supplying the lower limb.

A typical course of events is for the acute attack to begin with lumbago. After two or three days the focus of pain shifts from the back to the buttock or thigh, and as it does so the pain in the back lessens considerably. According to Cyriax (1982b), once this has happened the patient can be assured that he will recover within six months, counting from the time that the pain shifted its position, but with the proviso that the patient is less than 60 years old; if he is older, no such guarantee can be given.

In addition to pain, there may be other symptoms due to nerve root compression. These include weakness, loss of reflexes and areas of impaired sensation; there may also be autonomic disturbances. Most of these disappear as recovery occurs, but loss of the ankle jerk may be permanent.

The cause of most acute attacks of low back pain is unknown. Cyriax (1982c) holds that they are almost always due to prolapsed intervertebral discs but this is by no means universally accepted. For Travell and Simons, for example, the commonest cause is active TPs in the back muscles, and there are many other theories. Ideas about treatment are equally varied; they include rest, exercises, physiotherapy, traction, surgery, injection of substances to dissolve the disc material, and manipulation, as well as acupuncture and TENS.

Current ideas about the causes and treatment of *chronic* low back pain are, if possible, even more confusing. At one extreme there are those, like Cyriax, who attribute it almost entirely to intervertebral disc prolapse, while at the other extreme Melzack and Wall seem to favour the idea that in many cases, at least, the problem is one of 'pain memory'. And there are many other theories.

The whole situation is made more complicated by the influence of psychological factors. These are of course important in any kind of pain, but they seem to be specially prominent in low back pain. There is nothing surprising in the fact that a patient who suffers chronic pain for a long time may become obsessed with his disease and depressed by it, and this does indeed often happen. Probably no one can suffer prolonged pain without becoming at least in some ways a different person. However, the converse can also occur. There is a distinct tendency for various psychological disorders, especially depression, to focus on the back and sometimes to express themselves wholly in terms of back pain. This type of back pain is merely one aspect of the larger problem which the Americans call 'somatisation'. There seem to be many patients who for one reason or another do not experience unhappiness as a mental state but instead project it in physical symptoms. These symptoms may be of any kind but the lower back is a favourite site for them to appear. In many cases, of course, the picture is not clear-cut; it is seldom a question of either/or, but rather of recognising that a patient's back pain is probably the 'final common path' for a number of causes.

Acupuncture and the lower back
Acupuncture can certainly be useful in a number of cases of low back pain and sciatica. My own experience of using it is very largely in chronic pain, but it can also be used in acute pain provided this is not too severe. Very severe pain, however, will require strong analgesics to control it.

In examining the patient, particular attention should be paid to gait and posture. If there are signs of nerve root compression in the lower limbs this makes the chances of success with acupuncture less, though not negligible. It is important to keep in mind the distinction between root pain and referred pain (all root pain is referred pain, but not all referred pain is root pain). Referred pain, unlike root pain, does not make it less likely that acupuncture will succeed.

The examination of the patient carried out thus far is the same as would be made by any doctor. The acupuncturist, however, now goes on to make a careful search for TPs. The position in which the patient is placed for this purpose is important. It might seem natural to place the patient prone to examine her, but I find it is generally better to ask her to lie on each side alternately, the lower leg being straight and the upper one semi-flexed at the hip and knee (Fig. 6/3). This puts the back and hip muscles under moderate tension, which is desirable for detection of TPs. Sometimes it is an advantage to place a pillow under the lumbar spine in order to straighten it. In all cases, however, the patient should also be examined standing to give an idea of her spinal mobility and her posture.

In low back pain TPs may be found in the lumbar paraspinal muscles; in traditional acupuncture terms this is roughly B23 to B28. Deep pressure may be required to elicit these TPs. TPs are also commonly found over the sacro-iliac joints and in the gluteal regions. The most important muscles in this context are the pyriformis, which needs to be examined with firm deep pressure, perhaps using both hands with one finger pressing down on another; gluteus maximus, which causes mainly local pain; gluteus medius, which causes TPs in the region of the iliac crest; and gluteus minimus, TPs which can give rise to sciatica.

The quadratus lumborum muscle is very important in relation to back pain; it often contains active TPs, and one in particular tends to lie deeply in the angle between the sacrum and the ilium. Deep downward pressure is needed to reach this. Other TPs may be found in the sacrospinalis. They probably also occur in the psoas but this muscle is not accessible to needling.

If TPs are found in these areas they should be needled, usually with long (50mm) needles. An effort should be made to locate the TPs accurately; the patient will know when the TP is reached and as a rule teh chi (p. 49) will be obtained. If difficulty is experienced in hitting the TP it can sometimes be activated by twirling the needle; twirling is done at first gently and then increasingly strongly until an effect is achieved. Throughout this treatment it is essential to watch the patient's face closely and to keep asking her what she is feeling. Some patients think they should maintain a stoical impassivity in the face of pain, so it is important to explain that one is relying on the feedback they provide to let one know where the needle point is.

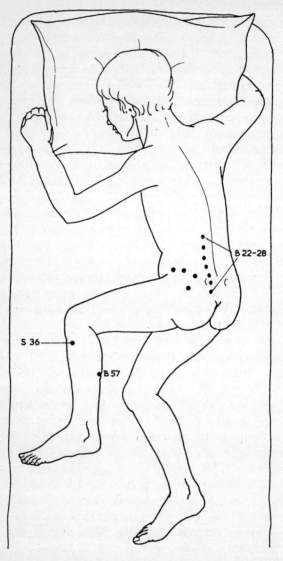

Fig. 6/3 Position of patients for examination and treatment. Also showing points B22–28; S36; B57

Some patients have large numbers of TPs throughout most of the spine. In such cases the best plan often seems to be to put in a number of needles (perhaps 8 or 10 pairs) fairly superficially along the whole length of the spine, with no particular attempt to needle individual TPs accurately. Superficial acupuncture of this kind also seems to be the best treatment for patients whose pain has a large psychological component. However, patients who complain of agonising pain in response to even light pressure should not receive acupuncture at all, since they will not be helped and will probably be made worse.

Periosteal acupuncture is also useful in low back pain. The laminae of the vertebral bodies from L2 to L5 may be needled; to do this, insert a 50mm needle about 2cm to one side of the midline, in a slightly medial direction, and advance the point until it strikes bone. The periosteum is then pecked in the usual way.

Another site for periosteal acupuncture is the neighbourhood of the sacro-iliac joint. The iliac crest can be felt and traced back to where it ends at the posterior superior iliac spine; the gap between the ilium and the sacrum can be felt below this. A 50mm needle inserted here will usually reach the bone. This is an interesting place to needle, because quite often the patient will experience sensations referred from the needle site as far down as the knee or even the foot. There is a tendency for these sensations to mimic or reproduce the pain habitually experienced by the patient, and if this occurs it is a good sign.

Periosteal acupuncture is usually the best treatment for sciatica. Acupuncture is unlikely to help Type C pain but it is often useful for Type A pain. In sciatica locally tender points may be found at various sites in the limbs below the gluteal region, but it is seldom a good idea to needle these, because as a rule it either does nothing or makes the patient worse.

Oddly enough, some patients who fail to respond to the treatments described so far may be helped by needling various points in the front of the abdomen. TPs may be found in the rectus abdominis muscles or the external oblique; Dr Macdonald (personal communication) suggests that the rectus TPs become more obvious if the patient is asked to raise her head against resistance while lying supine. If they are present these TPs should be needled using the superficial technique; if no TPs are found the abdominal wall can be needled in several places at random. Alternatively, periosteal needling can be carried out over the superior iliac spine.

Sciatica is one disorder in which it is worth while continuing to treat patients at intervals over a considerable period, perhaps several months, provided some improvement, no matter how modest, is occurring. I discovered this when I first started using acupuncture; a woman with severe sciatica, which she had had for several years, came for treatment. Acupuncture seemed to make little difference at first, so I admitted her to hospital for more frequent treatment. After about three weeks she was not much better, so I sent her home, telling her I did not think I could help her. However, she came back to see me, saying that she felt it was worth continuing for a time. I therefore went on treating her as an outpatient about every two weeks for about three months, after which she was almost cured. Some years later she sent a friend with a similar problem to see me, and I then learnt that she had not had a recurrence of her sciatica.

Acupuncture can occasionally be helpful in acute low back pain, even with sciatica, as well as in acute exacerbations of chronic low back pain, but owing to the kinds of patient who attend my clinics I have little experience of acute back problems. GV26, in the centre of the upper lip, is said to be effective in such cases, provided strong stimulation is used; strong stimulation at this point would be painful, and probably this is an example of diffuse noxious inhibitory control.

The hip
Pain in the hip may be referred from the spine or from TPs in the gluteal muscles, in which case these should be treated. However, the pain may also arise from the hip joint itself; typically this is due to osteoarthrosis, which will be confirmed radiologically. Considerable relief can often be achieved in such cases by periosteal needling of the greater trochanter of the femur; this is most easily carried out with the patient lying on her side with the affected hip uppermost. There may also be

TPs in the gluteal region, typically just behind the greater trochanter (G30). This treatment is a useful and safe alternative to anti-inflammatory drugs for patients who are awaiting a hip replacement.

The knee

The knee is one of the best joints to treat with acupuncture. As usual with joints, periosteal needling is the main standby, and regardless of where the pain is felt the medial aspect of the upper end of the tibia, where the bone is nearest the surface, is normally the site to use. This is often a TP but it can be used even if it is not tender. Treatment here is usually fairly painful and therefore need not be prolonged; 5–10 seconds is usually enough, and one treatment may give several weeks' or even months' relief.

A different kind of knee pain can occur acutely; it is not due to an internal derangement of the knee but appears to arise from the iliotibial tract close to its attachment to the femur on the lateral side of the knee. This is an example of a sports injury that can be treated very effectively with acupuncture.

Case study: While on a recent cycling tour in mountainous country I began to experience pain in the left knee. I first became aware of it while walking on the second day; by the third day it was worse and I began to think I might have to abandon the tour. The pain seemed to affect the whole knee though it was worse on the lateral side. Examining the knee, I found that there was an acutely tender TP over the lateral condyle of the femur; pressure here caused pain to radiate strongly over the knee. I always carry acupuncture needles with me on tour, and I therefore needled the TP. Next morning there was no pain; it recurred slightly during the morning's ride but then disappeared for the following week. On the penultimate day of the tour it returned, though not so severely; I sat down beside the road and needled the TP there and then. Within half an hour the pain had totally disappeared and it has never troubled me since.

It is important to remember that knee pain may be referred from a more proximal site. This may be the hip – pain in the knee referred from the hip is a well-known clinical phenomenon – but it may also be a muscle TP. In young patients particularly, there is often a TP in the vastus medialis at approximately the junction between the upper two-thirds and lower one-third of the thigh. In such cases the muscle TP should be treated as well as, or instead of, the medial aspect of the tibia.

The ankle and foot
Pain in these regions may be referred from proximal TPs; for example, in the peroneal muscles (S36) or posteriorly (B57). Pain in the heel is usually attributed to a calcaneal spur if one is found on the radiograph, but in many cases muscle TPs will exist, especially in the soleus. Non-specific pain in the ankle and foot often seems to respond quite well to non-specific periosteal needling, especially the talus, navicular and cuneiforms.

MAINTENANCE OF IMPROVEMENT

In chronic musculoskeletal disorders, pain and other symptoms will recur unless the factors that gave rise to the problem in the first place can be rectified. It is therefore necessary to take a careful history, with particular attention to habitual patterns of use that may be perpetuating the TPs. Driving and typing are two common causes of chronic musculoskeletal disorders; holding the body in a particular attitude for long periods appears to activate the TPs. Patients should be encouraged to change their position every half hour or so and to stretch their arms, shoulders, and neck. Recurrent neck and shoulder TPs due to faulty posture or psychological tension are a particularly common problem; it is often helpful for patients to ask their relatives to massage the shoulders and neck, which should be done using firm pressure so as to cause discomfort but not severe pain. Another useful trick is ice massage, which provides a strong cutaneous stimulus. A bag of frozen peas makes a convenient ice bag.

Travell and Simons (1983b; 1984c) provide numerous suggestions for stretching particular muscles to prevent recurrence of TPs and discuss the use of heel lifts to correct short legs and buttock lifts to correct a small hemipelvis. They believe that short upper arms are an important cause of TPs in the shoulders and that patients with this feature should have supports fitted to the arms of their chairs to prevent their shoulders from being dragged downwards.

SUMMARY

The treatment of musculoskeletal problems with acupuncture comes down mainly to the detection and treatment of TPs. This requires careful search and the TPs may be quite remote from the site of pain. However, it is possible to make certain generalisations.

As a rule, TPs refer pain forwards, downwards and distally, so in the first instance they should be sought near the spine and in the proximal regions of the limbs. TPs may also cause local pain in the area where they are located.

Distant acupuncture points are used relatively seldom, but can be valuable on occasion.

REFERENCES

Berry, H. et al (1980). Clinical study comparing acupuncture, physiotherapy, injections and oral anti-inflammatory drugs in shoulder cuff lesions. *Current Medical Research Opinion*, **7**, 121–6.

Bunker, T. D. (1985). Time for a new name for 'frozen shoulder'. *British Medical Journal*, **291**, 1233.

Camp, V. (1986). Acupuncture for shoulder pain. *Acupuncture in Medicine*, **3**, 28–32.

Cyriax, J. (1982a). *Textbook of Orthopaedic Medicine*, 8th edition, pp. 143–7. Baillière Tindall, London.

ibid. (1982b). p. 260.

ibid. (1982c). p. 221.

Mann, F. (1980). *The Treatment of Disease by Acupuncture*, pp. 194–6. Heinemann Books, London.

90 THE TREATMENT OF MUSCULOSKELETAL DISORDERS

O'Brien, J. P. (1984). In *A Textbook of Pain*, pp. 240–5, (eds. Wall, P. and Melzack, R.). Churchill Livingstone, Edinburgh.

Travell, J. G. and Simons, D. G. (1983a). *Myofascial Pain and Dysfunction*: *The Trigger Point Manual*, pp. 565–6. Williams and Wilkins, Baltimore.

ibid. (1983b). p. 196.

Travell, J. G. and Simons, D. G. (1984a). In *A Textbook of Pain*, p. 265, (eds. Wall, P. and Melzack, R.). Churchill Livingstone, Edinburgh.

ibid. (1984b). p. 264.

ibid. (1984c). p. 274.

Chapter Seven
OTHER DISORDERS

Many doctors who practise acupuncture part-time seem never to use it to treat anything except musculoskeletal disorders. This is a pity, because acupuncture can be effective in a number of diseases and symptom pictures that are not musculoskeletal, and in fact treatment of these 'other' disorders is one of the most fascinating and rewarding applications of acupuncture. There is, however, a good deal of overlap between the two groups and indeed in many cases treatment of so-called non-musculoskeletal disorders actually depends on the identification of TPs, so that the separation of the two groups is to some extent a descriptive convenience.

GENERAL CONSIDERATIONS

How should the treatment of these disorders be approached? The classic Chinese method, as we have seen, consists in using the traditional diagnostic techniques, especially the pulse, to decide which organs need tonifying or sedating and then to apply treatment to effect the required balance. Western doctors who do not use this system – and, it appears, a considerable number of modern Chinese acupuncturists as well – instead rely on 'cook books'. These are simply lists of acupuncture points to try in the treatment of a given disease or symptom picture. For example, a little book by the College of Chinese Medicine translated into English (Clausen, 1966) lists treatments for such things as colds, diarrhoea, epilepsy, insomnia, toothache, malaria, and so on.

If one studies the treatments recommended in such books, a pattern begins to emerge. The treatments depend on a combination of local and remote stimulation at named acupuncture points. The local points appear to be commonly encountered TPs in the vast majority of cases, while the remote points are usually chosen in accordance with channel theory: the channels on which they lie run through the affected area.

For example, in the book I have just mentioned the points listed for generalised headache are GV20, G20, GV16; LI 4, B54, and B60. The first three of these are local points which might well be active TPs in someone suffering from headaches, while the remaining three are distant points in the legs. Similarly, for stomach pain, including that due to gastric and duodenal ulcers, we find CV12, B18, B20, B21, P6, S36. The first four are local points, the last two distant.

It seems to me that the use of a cook book gives one the worst of both worlds. The traditional system, whether or not it is acceptable to a doctor who has received a modern scientific training, is at least rich and sophisticated and requires years of study to learn and apply, whereas the cook-book approach is routine and uninteresting. It has neither the scope of the traditional system nor the scientific basis of modern acupuncture and there is thus little to recommend it except its simplicity. And even this is not a real advantage, for if it fails there is nothing to fall back on. All the doctor can then do, if he still wants to treat his patient with acupuncture, is to try a different cook book; but as all the books tend to repeat the same information this is unlikely to help much.

A better approach, it seems to me, is to think about what one is doing in physiological and pathological terms as far as possible. This does not of course preclude the use of traditional ideas on occasion, but it does provide a broad and rational basis on which one can build.

In trying to decide on the treatment to use in a given case of non-musculoskeletal disorder, one should ask oneself the following questions:

1. Is this a TP disorder?

Many patients suffer from symptoms that are really due to TPs but are misdiagnosed as something else.

Case study: A man of 23 had suffered for several years from pain radiating from his left flank to his groin. This had at first been diagnosed as epididymitis but it failed to respond to antibiotics. He then saw a surgeon privately; an intravenous pyelogram was performed which did not show anything wrong, but apparently he nevertheless was told that he was suffering from kidney stones.

On examination he proved to have active TPs in his lumbar region and buttocks, and a few treatments to these relieved his symptoms. A complicating feature in this case was that the patient was suffering from the hyperventilation syndrome, which may have played a part in the perpetuation of his TPs. Correction of his breathing was needed in addition to acupuncture to achieve a full cure.

2. Is it something that might respond to generalised stimulation?

The question whether particular acupuncture points such as Liv3, S36, and LI 4 have specific effects as claimed in the classic Chinese literature is still unresolved, and I suspect likely to remain so for some time. It might seem a comparatively easy matter to satisfy oneself, at least, that such specific effects do or do not occur, but in fact it is very difficult. Sometimes, it is true, one does seem to see them, but very similar results can often also be achieved by needling 'incorrect' points, at least in some patients.

Provisionally, therefore, I think in terms of generalised but non-specific stimulation, and I regard the commonly used points such as Liv3, S36, and LI 4 as sites at which it is particularly easy to influence the functioning of the nervous, endocrine and possibly immune systems generally. This leaves open the question whether they have more specific effects over and above this.

Another uncertainty concerns the size of these points. Does one need to localise them very precisely, say within half a centimetre, or are they larger? Probably the answer to this question varies from patient to patient, but I think that in most cases they are at least a couple of centimetres in diameter. As we saw in Chapter 2, it may be possible to detect at least certain of the classic acupuncture points electrically, but whether this has any practical clinical significance is another question about which there is so far no evidence from research.

3. Is there an alternative acupuncture approach that might work?

One of the most interesting developments in acupuncture in the last few decades has been the application of modern ideas derived from scientific neurophysiology. Modern Chinese acupuncturists, for example, base a good deal of their treatment, not on the ancient theory of channels, but on modern knowledge of dermatomes. This is essentially the rationale for simple needling in the painful area. If one thinks about clinical problems in a neurological way one can sometimes devise new kinds of treatment not found in either the traditional texts or the cook books. A good example of this is transcutaneous electrical nerve stimulation (TENS), which, though similar to acupuncture in a number of ways, depends on ideas and technology that were not available to the ancients.

In this chapter I describe the treatments I have used for certain problems, and it might appear that I am in effect contradicting myself by first condemning the cook-book approach and then listing points to use in various circumstances. I want to emphasise, therefore, that the treatments I describe are primarily intended to illustrate the approach I am recommending and are not put forward as necessarily the right method to use in all circumstances. It is the general idea that matters rather than the exact details. Each patient is different and must be approached differently; moreover, each doctor will have a different kind of practice. The problems a general practitioner will encounter, for example, are not the same as those that confront an anaesthetist running a pain clinic. Again, if a doctor practises acupuncture full-time all his patients come expecting acupuncture and he will therefore find himself treating problems for which a general practitioner might not think of trying this form of treatment. Practising acupuncture full-time therefore naturally widens one's appreciation of the scope of the technique although at the same time it limits one's experience of general medicine, since there are many problems to which acupuncture has no application.

In my own case, most of the patients I see are suffering from long-term chronic or recurrent disorders and so I have comparatively little experience in the treatment of acute problems. For knowledge of the role of acupuncture in the treatment of acute disorders I have to rely largely on my reading and on the reports of colleagues who do see these things.

HEADACHE AND MIGRAINE

It is convenient to begin with headache, because the treatment is quite similar to that used for musculoskeletal neck and shoulder pain. From the acupuncture point of view there is not much need to distinguish between migraine and ordinary headache, and this agrees with a trend in modern medicine, for at least some neurologists are nowadays tending to the view that the two kinds of headache cannot be separated reliably.

Local treatment consists in needling any TPs that may be found in the shoulders, neck, or head. The common sites for these are G21, G20½, G20, and the temporalis muscles on either side of the temples. Ordinarily patients are treated on both sides at some or all of these points, the needles being inserted and usually twirled for between 30 seconds and 2 minutes.

General treatment consists in needling remote points, usually Liv3 and sometimes LI 4. Again, stimulation is usually given for between 30 seconds and 2 minutes on the first occasion, but, as always, the patient's response must be the guide. These remote points can be used as well as, or instead of, the local points.

The treatment I have just described is intended primarily as a prevention rather than as a cure for an existing headache, although it can also be used in acute attacks. However, the possibility of aggravations must always be kept in mind. On one

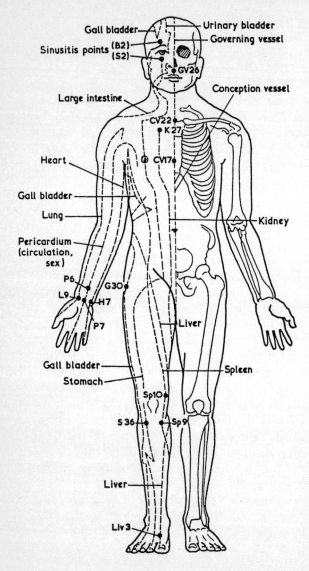

Fig. 7/1 The main points used – front view of the body

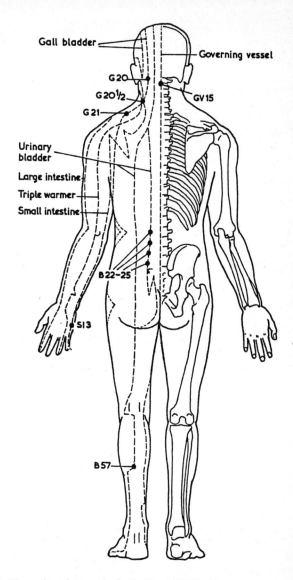

Fig. 7/1 The main points used – back view of the body

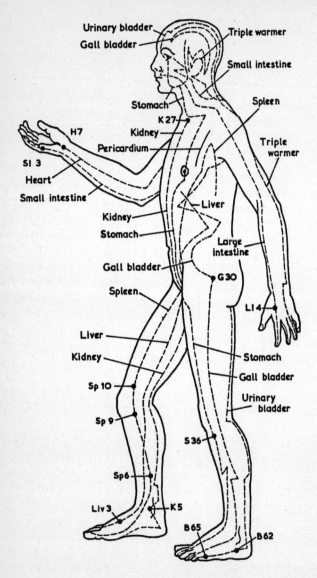

Fig. 7/1 The main points used – lateral view of the body

training course for doctors I followed my usual practice of getting all the participants to needle each other at LI 4 to allow them to experience the characteristic needle sensation. As I normally do, I asked if any of the doctors present thought they were likely to be strong reactors; none did, so I told them to carry on. Unfortunately, one woman doctor failed to mention that she had occasionally suffered from migraines. Had she done so I would have made sure that she was needled only lightly; as it turned out, that evening she suffered the worst migraine of her life and was unable to come to the course next day.

The results of acupuncture in headache are generally good; it is a Group A disorder. Some patients experience a reduction in the severity of the headaches, the frequency remaining more or less the same, while others find that the headaches become less frequent. Some patients find that the headaches now respond to analgesic drugs whereas before they were resistant.

The treatment is more likely to work when there are definite TPs in the neck; it does not seem to be less likely to work if the patient is depressed. However, cure is seldom total and most patients need to have further treatment at intervals of perhaps a few months.

An important point has emerged from a recent trial of acupuncture in headache which was carried out at the National Hospital for Nervous Diseases in London (Loh et al, 1984). In the report of this trial (which, incidentally, showed acupuncture to be clearly superior to medical treatment) we are told that two patients suffering from brain tumours (who were not in the trial) had headache that was relieved by acupuncture. The possibility that acupuncture may mask serious disease by relieving the symptoms temporarily must always be remembered.

The results in children suffering from migraine are outstandingly good; as a rule, a single treatment, with quick insertion of just one needle into Liv3 unilaterally, will give lasting relief to a child who may have been experiencing severe migraines as often as three times a week for years. I have now been able to follow up some of these children for up to nine years; they continue to gain good relief from acupuncture now that they are young adults, and come back for treatment perhaps once or twice a year.

A very interesting study of the long-term treatment of headache has recently been reported by Dr Seppo Junnila (1986) from Finland. He wrote to 121 patients who had been treated with acupuncture at a national health centre in south-west Finland; 115 replied. The length of follow-up was 2–4 years for 35 patients, 4–6 years for 15, 6–8 years for 36, and over 8 years for 29; thus more than half the patients were followed up for more than 6 years.

Treatment was always given by Dr Junnila. It was carried out on three to six occasions at intervals of one or two weeks initially, after which the patients were told to make another appointment if necessary.

Treatment was ineffective in 23 per cent of the patients. In 22 per cent there was a very considerable reduction in the frequency and severity of headache for over two years after a single course of treatment; mean pain reduction in this group was estimated at 81 per cent.

The third group (55 per cent) had a reduction in their headache which lasted on average 10 months.

Most studies of acupuncture in the treatment of headache have been based on a follow-up period of about six months. Dr Junnila's findings are thus exceptionally interesting, since it shows that the results of acupuncture are maintained over a long period, with treatment being repeated 3.3 times a year on average. It is difficult to dismiss results of this kind as due to placebo effect; and in fact the question whether acupuncture is a placebo in these circumstances largely loses its meaning.

Although migraine generally does well, another form of headache, which is in many ways similar, generally fails to respond, at least in my experience; this is cluster headache.

ATYPICAL MIGRAINE

Some patients suffer from attacks which may for convenience be described as atypical migraine, though whether they really

OTHER DISORDERS 101

are migrainous in nature is uncertain. The characteristic features of the attacks are that they are episodic, like migraine, and usually take the form of localised pain. For example, in one case there was recurrent pain in one ear; examination of this ear showed an acutely tender spot, and needling this (as well as Liv3) produced very good relief. In another case, there was a history of recurrent attacks of right-sided abdominal pain going back over many years. This had led to suspicion of gall stones, and in fact the patient's gall bladder had been removed without improvement. A course of acupuncture in the painful area and at Liv3 gave considerable improvement though not a complete cure.

OTHER NEUROLOGICAL PROBLEMS

There are some very interesting applications of acupuncture to other neurological problems.

Facial pain quite often responds, whether or not it has been diagnosed as trigeminal neuralgia. The treatment I currently use for this consists in deep needling in the region of the spheno-palatine ganglion; I learnt this from Dr A. Stephens, of Australia. The patient is placed lying on the side with the affected side uppermost. The needle is then inserted just below the zygomatic arch in front of the anterior ramus of the mandible and is inserted in a slightly upward and slightly backward direction to a depth of about three-quarters of an inch and left *in situ*, with or without stimulation, for one or two minutes. Usually one or two treatments are sufficient. It is important to study the anatomy of the region carefully before undertaking this treatment.

An alternative treatment for facial pain is simply to carry out superficial needling in the region of the affected division of the Vth cranial nerve. If the pain is very severe it is probably safer to start treatment on the opposite side.

Distant points that can be used include B62 and LI 4. I am not convinced that these add a great deal to the effectiveness of treatment.

Peripheral neuritis does not on the whole respond well to acupuncture, but pain due to diabetic neuropathy seems to be an exception. Liv3, B57, S36, and so on may be used, but in fact needling anywhere in the painful area seems to be effective. This is an example of the use of regional acupuncture.

Clonic facial spasm (facial myoclonia) is a disorder in which the patient suffers from twitching of one side of the face and spasm of the eyelid on that side. It is to be distinguished from blepharospasm, in which both eyes close tightly for long periods. The cause of the disorder is unknown, and there is no orthodox treatment. At first I had no success in treating it, but in the last few years I have had good results in a number of patients by needling the infra-orbital nerve where it emerges from the skull at the infra-orbital foramen. This can be felt under the orbit, but it is best not to insert the needle point into the foramen; it seems to be enough to needle the branches of the nerve as they spread out over the maxilla. I first used this technique on a patient for whom I had been trying other methods on and off for nearly a year, so in her case at least it was unlikely to have been a placebo response. I had treated this patient by needling the region of the facial nerve to start with, but this was only moderately successful. The patient herself noticed that needling closer to the eye worked better, and it then (somewhat belatedly) occurred to me that a more rational approach would be to apply the stimulus to the afferent arm of the arc. The results were gratifying: the twitching stopped as though a switch had been thrown, and it did not return for several hours. In this case I later went on to use TENS, but for subsequent patients I have used about six acupuncture treatments. Acupuncture usually stops the twitching immediately, though sometimes instead there is an immediate temporary increase; if acupuncture is repeated a few times at intervals the twitching is usually considerably diminished in frequency and intensity even if it is not totally abolished.

Writer's cramp is another disorder whose cause is unknown, though current opinion seems to favour the idea that it is not primarily psychological but is due to some abnormality of the way in which the brain controls movement. As a rule, acupuncture does not seem to work in writer's cramp, but I have seen a few patients in whom the difficulty in writing seems to be due, not to central causes in the brain, but to active TPs in the shoulders and forearm muscles; in these cases acupuncture is successful.

Carpal tunnel syndrome can quite often be helped by acupuncture. TPs should be sought in the neck and shoulders and also in the flexor muscles of the forearm. Acupuncture will not of course reverse severe changes such as wasting, but it is beneficial in cases of nocturnal pain and paraesthesiae. It seems possible that when this treatment is successful it works by reducing the accumulation of oedema fluid under the flexor retinaculum.

Vertigo, if mild, can sometimes be helped by acupuncture; the neck is the region to treat in these cases. Vertigo can have a number of causes, but in the patients who respond to acupuncture it is usually due to abnormal proprioceptive impulses arising from the facet joints in the neck. I think this is one of the commonest causes of vertigo in the elderly; it is much commoner than vertebrobasilar insufficiency, which is what is often diagnosed in such cases. Acupuncture is unlikely to help in vertigo due to Ménière's disease.

Tinnitus may conveniently be discussed here, though it is not really a neurological problem. Acupuncture has little or no effect in true tinnitus arising from a disturbance of the auditory nerve or inner ear. However, quite a number of patients who complain of 'tinnitus' are really suffering from something else; in some such cases, especially when there is a history of an injury to the neck or head, the cause seems to be TPs in the neck or head, and in these circumstances acupuncture can be curative. It is important, therefore, not to be put off treating a patient by the label that may have been attached to her problem but to reassess the situation for oneself.

PSYCHOLOGICAL DISORDERS

On the whole, acupuncture does not have a great deal of application to psychiatric problems; certainly not to the psychoses, but it can be useful in some cases of mild to moderate anxiety and depression. Traditionally the liver is supposed to be involved in depression, and Liv3 is therefore a point to try. For anxiety a number of points are given: P6, H7, and L9 at the front of the wrist and also GV15 and GV26. I am not myself convinced that most of these so-called tranquillising points have any marked effect in anxiety, and the only one I normally use (and that not very often) is GV15. This is situated over the atlanto-axial joint at the back of the neck, and some Chinese acupuncture tests have alarming diagrams showing insertion of needles here almost to the depth of the brainstem. This is of course not to be recommended, but gentle insertion to a depth of about 5mm, followed by gentle twirling for 2 or 3 minutes, is safe. In some people this does seem to have a definite tranquillising effect.

The most useful acupuncture method for tranquillising, however, seems to be to treat the TPs in the neck and shoulders (G21, G20½, G20) in just the same manner as one treats headaches. G21, in fact, appears in a great many cook-book 'recipes', perhaps because it is a useful tranquillising point and because psychological tension plays a part in the production or perpetuation of so many symptoms.

An interesting effect sometimes seen is emotional abreaction following needling of TPs in the shoulders or elsewhere. Patients occasionally laugh or cry uncontrollably for several hours after treatment. These effects are uncommon but interesting. They suggest that there is a reciprocal relationship between TPs and psychological tension. It seems possible that emotional stress can cause TPs to develop in muscle, and that the 'memory' of such stress is somehow locked up in these TPs; needling the TPs can bring the memory back into awareness. Similar reports have come from practitioners of other forms of physical treatment, such as Rolfing.

'ALLERGIC' DISORDERS

Allergic or presumed allergic disorders quite often respond to acupuncture. Ordinarily I use Liv3 for these, though I might on occasion add S36 or LI 4. The commonest of such disorders is recurrent urticaria (nettle rash), in which the patient suffers repeated attacks of itchy weals. These usually do well, although the duration of response is variable. This is one of the disorders in which it may be useful to teach the patient to treat herself.

There seems to be no good reason why patients should not practise self-acupuncture, provided they are willing to do so; after all, diabetic patients inject themselves with insulin daily for years without ill effects.

Case study: A 37-year-old man had suffered from almost continuous urticaria for a number of years. He responded quickly to acupuncture at Liv3; each treatment gave him several weeks' relief, but unfortunately repeated treatments did not greatly prolong the duration of relief. He was therefore taught to needle himself at Liv3, which he did every two or three weeks. This worked well and he has had no further problems.

In some cases, if not in all, chronic or recurrent urticaria is due to a food sensitivity or allergy, and this should be sought and identified if possible. Often, however, it is not possible. In any case, allergy is seldom an all-or-nothing affair, and most doctors practising acupuncture gain the impression that treating patients in this way can sometimes abolish or at least diminish specific allergies.

Some patients suffer from symptoms that are probably not allergic but for which there is no obvious explanation. Some of these do very well with acupuncture.

Case study: A 45-year-old woman had suffered for five years from recurrent attacks of diarrhoea associated with bleeding. This sounded like ulcerative colitis but investigation of the bowel did not show any cause for her symptoms. A curious feature of the diarrhoea was that it occurred only during the winter, lasting for six months at a time. In addition, she was subject to solar urticaria: if she went out into the sun even for a short time she suffered an outbreak of itchy weals. In spite of very intensive tests no cause had been found for her symptoms and no treatment could be offered. After a course of acupuncture, however, the problem was largely resolved: she no longer suffered diarrhoea in winter and she could stand at least moderate exposure to sunlight without ill-effects.

Mysterious disorders of this kind, for which no one has managed to find an orthodox diagnosis, but which do not seem to be primarily psychological, are among the most rewarding problems to treat with acupuncture. It is impossible to list all the kinds of symptom that may fall into this category, because by definition they are anomalous and unpredictable; but, in general terms, one should keep acupuncture in mind whenever one encounters symptoms or groups of symptoms that are episodic, recurring at intervals of weeks or perhaps months, in a patient who does not seem to be neurotic (even though she may well have been told that the problem is psychological at some time in the past). In such cases one should make a careful search for TPs; if none is found, try 'non-specific' treatment by needling Liv3 and perhaps LI 4 or S36 as well.

In traditional Chinese medicine the liver is supposed to be responsible for certain rather ill-defined symptoms including fatigue, mild nausea, dislike of fatty foods, and a general non-specific malaise; the picture is rather like that of a mild hangover. (Curiously enough, the French also attribute such symptoms to the liver. Most British doctors would tend to dismiss patients with complaints of this kind as neurotic.)

Whatever the cause of these symptoms, they often respond remarkably well to acupuncture, the needles usually being inserted at Liv3. Patients with these complaints often spontaneously report a clearing of their vision immediately after acupuncture.

The *post-viral syndrome* can conveniently be considered here. A number of patients experience fatigue, muscular aching, and vague recurrent malaise for months or even years after a presumed viral infection. That these effects can follow an attack of infectious mononucleosis (glandular fever) is well known, but there is some evidence that they can also be produced by other viral infections, though this is difficult to prove and the importance of psychological factors in any individual case is hard to determine. Acupuncture is certainly worth trying in such cases and sometimes works well. Liv3, once again, is probably the best point to try, although I usually use S36 as well in view of its supposed stimulatory effects on the immune system.

NAUSEA AND VOMITING

At the Queen's University of Belfast Professor J. W. Dundee (1986) and his colleagues have recently carried out two consecutive studies in which acupuncture at P6 was used as an anti-emetic in patients receiving premedication before gynaeco-logical operations. Two control groups were used: one of these received premedication alone, while the other received premedication plus acupuncture at an 'incorrect' site. The patients given 'real' acupuncture experienced significantly less nausea than those in either of the control groups; 'dummy' acupuncture did not reduce the incidence of nausea.

Another anaesthetist, Dr E. N. S. Fry (1986), has treated 500 postoperative patients with 'acupressure', performed by pressing 'with the flat of three fingers over the flexor aspect of either wrist over and just proximal to the skin creases for half a minute with force equivalent to a firm handshake'. Eleven patients in the treated group were sick compared with 40 in the control group.

Both authors think that such treatments are worth trying as a preventive for nausea and vomiting in pregnancy.

RESPIRATORY PROBLEMS

Rhinitis: Patients who suffer from early morning sneezing and, to a lesser extent, other symptoms of 'chronic sinusitis' such as a blocked nose and nasal discharge, can sometimes be helped with acupuncture. The treatment I usually try is periosteal needling over the frontal and maxillary sinuses (approximately B2 and S3, but the exact location is not important). This treatment will produce an immediate clearing of the nose in almost every patient who suffers from nasal obstruction, and if it is repeated on a few occasions there may be prolonged relief. If this treatment fails it is worth trying needling the region of the sphenopalatine ganglion, as described for facial pain (p. 101).

Case study: A 42-year-old man had suffered from severe attacks of paroxysmal sneezing for 10 years; conventional treatment, including nasal corticosteroid sprays, had failed to help him. He was treated with periosteal needling to the sinuses. On the first occasion the immediate effect was an outbreak of violent sneezing, and this occurred again, although less violently, on the next few occasions. After four treatments he was symptom free and remained so for several months. He then relapsed although not to his former condition; another course of treatment once more abolished his sneezing.

Hay fever: A specific form of rhinitis due to allergy to pollen. From the acupuncture point of view this is a B disorder; it can be helped in a third to a half of patients. The sinuses or the sphenopalatine region may be treated in the manner just described for rhinitis, but Liv3 should always be included. In the best cases a single treatment will prevent hay fever symptoms occurring throughout the whole season, but more commonly a number of treatments will be required. This is another of the disorders in which it may be useful to teach patients to treat themselves if relief lasts only a short time.

Asthma: Acupuncture treatment is often described and might be expected to give good results and is mentioned in cook books, but I have not myself found it to be very effective; I would not rate it higher than C. *Local* treatment consists in needling the chest wall; specific points include CV17, CV22, G21, and B11-B18. Remote points to try are Liv3 and LI 4. It is important to treat asthmatic patients carefully, since there is a possibility of causing a severe aggravation if stimulation is too vigorous.

If an asthmatic patient's lung function is monitored using a peak flow meter before and after acupuncture it is sometimes possible to demonstrate an immediate improvement, but equally there may also be an actual deterioration even though the patient feels better subjectively. Much the same applies to the long-term effects; patients may feel that their breathing is better even though there is no objective change in performance. I therefore tend to think that, in many cases, acupuncture works merely as a placebo in asthma.

In spite of these rather negative comments, however, small numbers of asthmatic patients do respond well.

Case study: A 47-year-old woman had suffered from seasonal asthma every summer for many years. A single treatment at Liv3 unilaterally at the beginning of summer prevented asthmatic attacks for the remainder of the year. The treatment was repeated every year for the next three years with the same satisfactory outcome.

GYNAECOLOGICAL DISORDERS

This is a fruitful field for acupuncture treatment. In traditional acupuncture certain points (Sp6, Sp9, Sp10) are supposed to be particularly related to gynaecological problems, and in fact these points, especially Sp6, do seem to become abnormally tender in such cases and may be regarded as TPs. Treatment of gynaecological disorders therefore consists in needling these points at the site of maximum tenderness. In addition, subcutaneous needling may be carried out over the lower abdomen and the corresponding area on the back (B22–B28).

This treatment gives very good results in dysmenorrhoea (A) and can also help some 30–50 per cent of patients suffering from other painful disorders such as pelvic inflammatory disease and endometriosis. Menorrhagia can also be improved. Patients suffering from amenorrhoea of recent onset can also be helped, though this disorder often recovers spontaneously and it is difficult to know how far acupuncture contributes to the outcome.

Premenstrual tension is a difficult problem, in which there is usually a complex mixture of physical and emotional factors; the role of acupuncture is correspondingly uncertain.

Menopausal symptoms, especially hot flushes, can be helped in about half the cases; Liv3 usually gives the best results here.

The traditional point used for *female sterility* is K5. There is no good research evidence to show that this treatment works, but there seems no *a priori* reason why acupuncture should not stimulate ovulation via an effect on the hypothalamus. For what it is worth, I have seen two patients who were being treated for unrelated problems who also, incidentally, had difficulties in conceiving, who became pregnant during treatment. If one does choose to try acupuncture as a treatment for sterility, it is important to remember the risk that it can also cause abortion; treatment should therefore be confined to the first half of the menstrual cycle.

GASTRO-INTESTINAL DISORDERS

Hiccough can be effectively treated, if there is no underlying pathology, by acupuncture to the epigastrium (whether or not there is a TP here).

Epigastric pain can likewise be treated by epigastric needling; usually there is an area of epigastric tenderness in such patients and this should be treated. This treatment is particularly suitable for patients who experience pain like that which occurs in peptic ulcer although investigations fail to reveal an ulcer; it can also be used when there is an actual ulcer, though whether it helps to heal the ulcer in such cases is doubtful. A distant point (S36) is traditionally used in such cases but I have not been able to convince myself that it makes much difference.

The dumping syndrome which may follow partial gastrectomy for peptic ulceration can sometimes be effectively treated with acupuncture. I have usually used Liv3, with or without S36, for this.

Case study: A man aged 42 had suffered from the dumping syndrome for several years following a partial gastrectomy. Acupuncture at Liv3 relieved his symptoms but only for about five days after each treatment. As he lived a long way from the hospital he was admitted for an intensive course of treatment in the hope that this would produce a more prolonged remission. However, the duration of remission was not increased. It then emerged that his wife was a nurse. She was therefore brought to the hospital and taught how to needle her husband, which she continued to do every five days or so following his discharge. Some nine months later he was being satisfactorily maintained symptom free on this treatment.

Ulcerative colitis, if not too severe, can be helped in some patients (B). The needles are usually inserted at Liv3 and locally, over the lower abdomen. The effect is greatest on pain; diarrhoea responds less well. The same treatment can be used for *diverticulosis* which can respond surprisingly well.

Case study: A 45-year-old man attended hospital for treatment of his diverticulosis, which was exceptionally severe; he had already had surgery for it but was continuing to experience severe unremitting pain. The symptoms had been present for 20 years. He did not come expecting acupuncture but readily agreed to try it; he quickly proved to be a quite exceptionally strong reactor. Within two minutes of the needles being inserted into his lower abdomen and Liv3 bilaterally he felt drowsy and ecstatic and his pain vanished; moreover, he remained free from pain for the next six weeks. Further treatments brought the duration of remission up to about three months, and he has continued to respond in the same way for four years. Each time he is treated he experiences the same ecstatic euphoria, which lasts for several hours afterwards, and the pain declines to negligible levels for many weeks.

This patient has described the immediate effects of treatment as follows: 'The minute the needles are inserted I become sleepy and immediately free from pain. The needles are left in for approximately 5–10 minutes. During that time I feel great and only wish it could last for ever.' After treatment, he writes, 'I have a feeling of well-being. The only side-effect is tiredness, which lasts most of the day. After a good night's rest I wake up refreshed and free from pain, which to me is heaven.'

CARDIOVASCULAR DISORDERS

There are relatively few applications of acupuncture in this field. The principle one is intermittent claudication, which responds well (A). The main point to use is B57; one treatment here can give weeks or even months of relief, with improvement in walking distance. The same treatment can be used in other types of vascular disease of the legs, whatever the cause, and for nocturnal cramps. An important self-help exercise for the patient suffering from night cramps is to stretch the calf muscles. To do this, place one foot behind the other and lean forward with the hands against a wall and the rearmost knee straight; the exercise is then repeated for the opposite leg.

Raynaud's disease seems to respond moderately well (B); if the hands are affected one can use GV14, with perhaps LI 4 as well. For the feet one stimulates the sacrum and also Liv3 and perhaps B57. (See Chapter 8 as well for a discussion of TENS in the treatment of Raynaud's disease.)

'Palpitations' is a term that patients may use to describe a wide range of cardiac irregularities as well as subjective awareness of a fast heart rate due to anxiety. Of the irregularities of rhythm, only frequent ectopic beats (if they trouble the patient) and paroxysmal tachycardia are worth considering for acupuncture treatment. The traditionally recommended points are H7 and K27. Travell and Simons (1983), in their book on TPs, describe a TP in the pectoralis major muscle in the 5th right interspace which they claim gives rise to paroxysmal tachycardia. I have not been able to confirm this myself so far but it is worth looking for and treating if found.

There are no convincing reports of the use of acupuncture to treat hypertension. In so far as it works at all it is probably the result of combined suggestion and relaxation.

SKIN DISORDERS

Here again the scope of acupuncture is limited. It can sometimes relieve itching in *eczema* but does not seem to have much effect on the rash. Traditionally the Lung points are used to treat skin diseases, but in practice it does not seem to make much difference where the needles are inserted, and the effect of acupuncture in eczema, if any, must therefore be non-specific.

The recurrence rate in *Herpes simplex* (both Type I and Type II) can sometimes be reduced by acupuncture, using Liv3. This, however, only seems to work in fairly strong reactors.

Psoriasis on the whole does not respond, though I have seen a few patients whose psoriasis cleared up after many years while they were being treated for other things; again, the exact points used do not seem to be important. Some acupuncturists treat localised areas of psoriasis by placing needles around it.

Post-herpetic neuralgia is a distressing problem that unfortunately does not respond to acupuncture, at least in my experience. However, it can sometimes be relieved by TENS (see Chapter 9).

MISCELLANEOUS PROBLEMS

Pain due to cancer

It is important to realise that the mere fact that a patient has cancer does not mean that any pain he may suffer is necessarily due to cancer. Such people may have musculoskeletal pain just like anyone else, so the importance of accurate diagnosis is particularly important in such cases. Musculoskeletal pain in cancer patients can of course be treated by acupuncture.

Acupuncture does have a limited role in the treatment of pain due to cancer, though there have been few reports of its use in such cases. Dr J. Filshie, an anaesthetist working in a pain clinic at the Royal Marsden Hospital, has assessed the effect of acupuncture in 183 out of 300 consecutive patients (Filshie and Redmond, 1986). (Those who were very ill or who had had nerve blocks were excluded.) She found that her early results were excellent: 82 per cent of the patients were helped for hours or days, but only 52 per cent obtained lasting benefit, and they often required repeated treatments. Acupuncture was most helpful for vascular problems, muscle spasm and disordered sensation, but it did also benefit a number of patients whose pain was directly due to their cancer. When these latter patients ceased to respond to acupuncture it was often a sign that their disease had worsened.

Acupuncture sometimes appears to reduce oedema of the arm due to surgery for breast cancer.

Phantom limb pain

The acupuncture treatment of this problem consists in needling the opposite limb. It can be effective, though an alternative approach depends on the use of TENS, to be discussed in Chapter 8.

LOCATION OF MAIN ACUPUNCTURE POINTS REFERRED TO IN THIS CHAPTER

G20, G20½, G21: See Chapter 6.

GV14: Over the spine of C7.

GV15: Opposite the atlanto-axial joint.

GV21: In the centre of the upper lip.

CV17: In the midline of the sternum, at the junction between the body of the sternum and the xiphoid process. Because the bone is very near the surface here, the needle must be inserted parallel to the skin in an upward direction.

CV22: In the jugular notch, between the clavicles. Some Chinese texts show a long needle being inserted behind the sternum to an alarming depth; this, needless to say, should not be done.

K5: Just behind the medial malleolus of the tibia.

K27: At the inner end of the clavicle. Here, again, the needle must be inserted almost parallel to the skin owing to the thinness of the tissues.

P6: On the front of the waist, 2 finger-breadths above the distal skin crease.

LI 4: On the dorsum of the hand in the middle of the web between the first and second metacarpals.

SI 3: At the ulnar side of the hand, opposite the neck of the fifth metacarpal. The needle should be inserted through the relatively thin skin at the edge of the hand, and not through the thicker (and more painful) palmar skin.

S36: On the outer side of the leg, over the neck of the fibula.

Sp6: About a handsbreadth above the medial malleolus of the tibia.

Sp9: On the medial side of the knee just below the medial condyle of the tibia.

Sp10: On the medial side of the knee just above the medial condyle of the femur.

B57: In the middle of the calf, between the two bellies of the gastrocnemius, where this muscle becomes tendinous. This site will often become more apparent if the patient is asked to stand on tiptoe.

B62: At the side of the heel, directly below the tip of the lateral malleolus of the tibia. The needle is passed beneath the calcaneum towards the medial side.

B65: Below the neck of the fifth metatarsal; the needle is passed medially from the lateral side.

Liv3: Between the first and second metatarsal bones, in the first dorsal interosseus muscle. The needle is inserted perpendicularly to a depth of about 12.5mm ($\frac{1}{2}$ inch).

REFERENCES

Clausen, T. (ed.) (1966). *Practical Acupuncture*. FADL Publishing House, Copenhagen.

Dundee, J. W. et al (1986). Traditional Chinese acupuncture: a potentially useful antiemetic? *British Medical Journal*, **293**, 583–4.

Filshie, J. and Redmond, D. (1986). Acupuncture for malignant pain problems. (Paper presented at the Second World Congress of Scientific Acupuncture, London.)

Fry, E. N. S. (1986). Antiemetic action of acupressure. (Points.) *British Medical Journal*, **292**, 1398.

Junnila, S.Y.T. (1986). Acupuncture for long time treatment of headache in National Health Centres. (Paper presented at the Second World Congress of Scientific Acupuncture, London.)

Loh, L. et al (1984). Acupuncture versus medical treatment for migraine and muscle tension headaches. *Journal of Neurology, Neurosurgery and Psychiatry*, **47**, 333–7.

Travell, J. G. and Simons, D. G. (1983). *Myofascial Pain and Dysfunction: The Trigger Point Manual*, p. 577. Williams and Wilkins, Baltimore.

Chapter Eight
ELECTRO-ACUPUNCTURE AND OTHER SPECIALISED TECHNIQUES

So far in this book I have said very little about electrical methods of acupuncture. This is because, with the notable exception of transcutaneous nerve stimulation (TENS), to be discussed in Chapter 9, I do not find electrical acupuncture to be very useful. However, it is necessary to say something about it, if only because the newcomer to acupuncture is likely to find himself bombarded by enticements to buy complicated machinery some of which may cost several hundreds or even thousands of pounds.

Electricity has been applied to acupuncture in two main ways: for treatment and for 'point diagnosis'.

Point diagnosis
This implies, of course, that one believes that there are such things as 'acupuncture points' in the first place. A great deal of ingenuity has been applied to the electrical detection of these points, and many machines are available commercially for the purpose. Nearly all rely on measurement of the resistance of the skin to passage of a current. It is usually claimed that acupuncture points possess a decreased (sometimes an increased) resistance. The difficulty is, however, that most of the machines sold for measuring resistance produce false readings (artefacts) with great readiness. Leaving the measuring probe in contact with the skin for a little longer than usual,

or pressing a little harder than usual, will produce an erroneus result. Moreover, repeated application of currents to the skin alters its resistance. There is thus a considerable tendency for the experimenter to produce 'acupuncture points' wherever he thinks they ought to be. Most scientific attempts to study the question have failed to confirm the reality of 'points'.

There are, however, one or two interesting exceptions. Reichmanis and Becker (1976) carried out one study at Upstate Medical Center, Syracuse, New York. The measuring electrode assembly consisted of 36 steel rods in a square of 6 rods × 6 rods connected to a DC Wheatstone bridge circuit. Using this rather elaborate apparatus, the researchers were able to demonstrate local variations in conductance at a number of classical acupuncture points on the Triple Warmer and Lung channels, though not all the points were detected in every subject.

Some researchers at the University of Missouri School of Medicine used a device that did not apply a current to the skin but instead measured the electrical activity of the body itself (Brown et al, 1974). The outer surface of the skin is electrically negative with respect to subcutaneous tissue, and the experimenters used this fact to test for acupuncture points. They found 18 points on the upper arm, which included all those shown as acupuncture points on charts as well as a few not shown. These points were distributed symmetrically on the two arms and did not change in situation or electrical activity over time.

At a more practical level, the most useful machine for detecting local electrical differences seems to be a Japanese device called the Neurometer. Provided this is used carefully it will pick out certain sites in every subject quite reproducibly. For example, I have never failed to find a pair of points at the back of the head, almost but not quite corresponding in position to G20 on the acupuncture charts. Constant points of this kind can also be found on the ear and probably elsewhere. What is interesting about them is that they are very small, probably about a millimetre in diameter. Sometimes the passage of the electrical current through them produces a pricking sensation.

Other kinds of point can also be detected with this machine. For example, areas of decreased impedance can be found on the back, though they are not as sharply demarcated as those on the ear or G20. There seems to be a tendency for these back areas to become more obvious when there are active TPs.

The significance of these electrically active areas is uncertain. Needham and Gwei-Djen (1980), in *Celestial Lancets*, report a convincing demonstration of many acupuncture points with the Neurometer; moreover, these points could still be demonstrated on a cadaver several hours after death. A Canadian acupuncturist, Dr C. Chan Gunn, who believes that many acupuncture points are muscle motor points, finds that the Neurometer can be used to detect them. He defines a muscle motor point as the site at which a muscle twitch can be elicited using the minimum electrical stimulus.

From the purely practical point of view I do not find any need to use electrical methods of point detection. For TPs I think it is preferable to rely on simple manual examination, while I do not think there is sufficient evidence for the clinical importance of classic acupuncture points to make it worth while spending time on attempting to detect them electrically.

Electrical stimulation
Electrical methods of stimulating acupuncture needles have been used for a number of years. The usual apparatus is a battery-powered machine that allows current to be fed to several pairs of needles at the same time. Direct current is unsuitable for this purpose because it weakens the needles owing to electrolytic effects; various kinds of biphasic current are therefore employed.

In my view electrical stimulation has little practical application to ordinary acupuncture, at least for the present. About the only use I have found for electrical stimulation in the past has been to treat large areas, for example in post-herpetic neuralgia; in such cases one may put several needles on each side of the painful area and pass a current between the opposed pairs. However, I am not myself convinced that the electrical stimulation actually does anything that is not achieved simply by the needles, without using any electricity. Moreover, it is rather an arbitrary kind of stimulus; manual stimulation, in contrast, can be precisely graded to the patient's response and is therefore a more sensitive tool.

More recently, I have experimented with a technique first suggested to me by Dr Macdonald in which large muscle groups (typically those in the anterior compartment of the leg) are stimulated strongly at 4Hz for about two minutes; one needle is inserted at S36 and the other at a random point distally. This method has given promising results in hay fever and the post-viral syndrome and it seems worth exploring further.

LASER THERAPY

Perhaps inevitably, the last few years have witnessed the production of various laser machines for acupuncture. It is claimed that these machines are as good as, or even better than, needles for stimulating acupuncture points, and have the advantage that they are painless and therefore suitable for use on children and people who are frightened of acupuncture. It is still too early to say whether these claims are valid, though Professor Johannes Bischko, head of the Ludwig Boltzmann Acupuncture Institute in Vienna, is enthusiastic about laser acupuncture and has carried out a number of experiments with it. What is certain is that the equipment is very expensive, and it seems prudent to wait at least for a time before moving into this new field.

EAR ACUPUNCTURE

The idea of using the external ear for acupuncture is largely due to a French doctor, Paul Nogier, of Lyon (see Kenyon, 1983a). In the early 1950s Nogier was intrigued to find that some of his patients had apparently been cured of their sciatica by a lay practitioner who had cauterised an area on their ears. On looking further into the matter, he found that this form of treatment had been used in France during the nineteenth century but had largely died out by 1870. Intrigued, he began to search the ears of patients who were suffering from various kinds of pain. Eventually he came to the conclusion that there is a map or representation of the body in the ear; the body is supposed to be represented upside down in a fetal position, with the head on the ear lobe and the spine on the ridge of the ear known as the anti-helix (Fig. 8/1). This will recall the representation of the body in the motor cortex of the brain that was first described by Wilder Penfield.

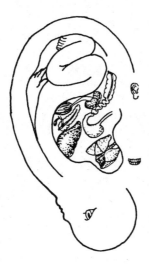

Fig. 8/1 The reversed homunculus superimposed on the ear

It seems that the mediaeval Chinese had also recognised the existence of acupuncture points in the ear but without describing an inverted homunculus. However, Nogier's charts were soon adopted in China, and before long translated versions of *their* translations of Nogier's charts began to appear in the West. Thus we now have at least two sets of ear charts: Nogier's, and Chinese charts probably based to a greater or lesser extent on Nogier's. There are quite a few discrepancies between these two versions.

Very few attempts have been made to investigate Nogier's claims objectively. Melzack (1984) tried, but failed, to find evidence for the specific correlations described by Nogier. On the other hand, researchers at UCLA School of Medicine have found such evidence (Oleson et al, 1980). Forty patients suffering from musculoskeletal pain in various parts of their bodies were tested. They were draped with a sheet to conceal any visible physical problems, and then a doctor who knew nothing about their illness examined their ears for areas of increased electrical conductance or tenderness. A correct identification was obtained in 361 out of 480 individual comparisons (75.2 per cent). There were 12.9 per cent false positive points (that is, 'reactive' ear points that did not correspond to areas of musculoskeletal pain), and 11.9 per cent false negative points ('non-reactive' points that did represent areas of musculoskeletal pain).

This is an interesting study, and its results are striking enough to prevent one's dismissing the idea of an ear representation of the body out of hand. Implausible though the notion may seem at first glance, the ear does have an exceptionally complicated nerve supply (greater auricular branch of the cervical plexus, lesser occipital nerve, auricular branch of the vagus and auriculotemporal nerve). It is therefore at least conceivable that the ear is connected with centres in several different parts of the brain and thus with remote parts of the body.

While this fact – if it is a fact – would certainly be of great interest to neuroanatomists, would it have any practical importance for doctors? The authors of the study believe that it would not help very much in diagnosis, since generally it would be easier simply to ask patients where they felt pain. However, it could be useful for unconscious patients or children. They also found that some patients who were told of the findings of the ear examination suddenly remembered previously forgotten pains or problems in the relevant area, and they therefore suggest that ear diagnosis could be useful in the general assessment of a patient.

The main claim made on behalf of Nogier's work, however, is that it is an effective method of treatment. When a reactive point is found in the ear, this is treated by needling and sometimes with electrical stimulation of the needle. Nogier has in fact developed a complete sub-system of acupuncture based on the ear. Moreover, he has moved on considerably from the simple initial method of examining the ear for tender points. He has designed a number of electrical instruments for detecting points in the ear, and in 1966 he described the 'auricular cardiac reflex' (see Kenyon, 1983b): that is, changes in the amplitude of the radial pulse in response to various stimuli. Perhaps the most startling of his ideas concerns the use of coloured filters which are applied to the skin of the ear; different colours are said to have varying effects on the pulse.

Much of this undoubtedly sounds strange to most Western doctors, and only a minority of medical acupuncturists have taken up Nogier's methods. One problem with ear acupuncture, which is admitted even by its advocates, is that relief of pain, if it occurs, often lasts for only a short time. Semipermanent needles are sometimes inserted in the ear and left in place for about seven days in an attempt to make the effect more lasting, but, as noted in Chapter 4, this is not entirely desirable in view of the risk of infection.

Ear acupuncture is used by some practitioners to treat obesity and smoking. The patient may be treated weekly, or a semipermanent needle may be inserted and the patient is instructed to press it whenever she feels the urge to eat or smoke, as the case may be. There is no evidence that acupuncture has more than a placebo effect in problems of this kind.

I have not myself used ear acupuncture a great deal but at times it can be useful, as the following case shows.

Case study: A married woman aged 30 attended the Royal London Homoeopathic Hospital with a history of five years' abdominal pain following an appendicectomy that had been complicated by peritonitis. The pain had been present almost continuously since then; it was situated in the right groin and radiated across the lower abdomen to the left. Sometimes it was stabbing, sometimes colicky. When it was severe she would vomit.

Since her initial appendicectomy she had had no fewer than 10 operations to relieve her pain, without improvement. A large number of diagnostic tests had been carried out, but nothing was found. She was given a TENS machine, which helped to some extent, but she continued to have pain. She did not respond to homoeopathy and was admitted to hospital in a severe attack; she was writhing with pain and obtained no relief from opioid drugs.

Local acupuncture to her abdomen did not help her at all. However, she proved to have a tender area in the margin of her right ear (that is, on the same side as the pain), and inserting a needle here produced an immediate cessation of her pain. She said she could feel a sensation as if the pain were about to come on but it did not actually do so.

At first the relief was very temporary; it lasted while the needle was in place but the pain returned as soon as stimulation was stopped. Electrical stimulation was therefore used to give a prolonged effect, and a gradual improvement followed. When she was discharged from hospital she continued to apply electrical stimulation to her ear via an inverted drawing pin fixed in position with a piece of tape; since the skin was unbroken there was no danger of infection and she continued the stimulation at intervals. Five months later she was still pain free, for the first time in five years.

Ear acupuncture is, I believe, worth remembering in any difficult case. It may not help often but, as the case just described illustrates, it can be very valuable. In keeping with my predilection for simple methods in acupuncture I do not use elaborate techniques for finding points. The ears should be searched on both surfaces for tender areas. Special spring-loaded probes are sold for the purpose but an exhausted ballpoint pen costs nothing and is just as good. (Indeed, this is a good instrument for searching for TPs anywhere, and not just in the ears.) The blunt end is used first for rough location of the tender point or points, and the pointed end is then used to allow more precision. There is no need to use charts either; one may take Nogier's inverted homunculus as a guide if this idea appeals, but the whole ear should in any case be searched.

If a TP is found in the ear it should be needled without piercing the cartilage, using a small fine needle (30mm, or 15mm if available). Needling the ear is fairly painful, for which reason a number of acupuncturists use lasers instead.

If the treatment works, it is likely to do so immediately, but as already noted improvement may well be only temporary. In that case one can try daily treatment for a time or apply a TENS machine to a semi-permanent electrode, such as the inverted drawing pin fixed in place with a piece of tape mentioned in the case described above. (The lead from the TENS machine must be fitted with a crocodile clip to attach to the electrode.)

ACUPUNCTURE ANALGESIA

Although it was acupuncture analgesia that first attracted the attention of the West in the current wave of interest, it has been relatively little investigated outside China. It now appears that some of the early claims for acupuncture analgesia were exaggerated: only a few patients (probably all strong reactors) are considered suitable for it and it works well only for certain kinds of operation. Patients may receive orthodox premedication in addition.

One does sometimes see analgesia in patients who are receiving routine acupuncture treatment. In one case, for example, a patient reported that whenever a needle was put into her foot at Liv3 she experienced a sensation in her gums as if she had had a local anaesthetic; and sure enough, when her gums were pricked with a needle she felt no pain. Another patient became insensitive to needling in the whole upper half of her body whenever a needle was inserted in Liv3.

Acupuncture analgesia has been used for selected patients in this country, but only to a very limited extent.

OTHER CHINESE INNOVATIONS

Although acupuncture is an ancient technique it is still very much alive and developing in its homeland, China, as well as elsewhere. The Chinese have, for example, introduced the practice of injecting vitamins, antibiotics, placental extracts, and extracts of herbal medicines at acupuncture points. They have also tried 'strong stimulation' at points where pain or tenderness is felt, including the actual 'massage' of principal peripheral nerves with forceps. Scalp acupuncture is still another new technique, which is claimed to stimulate the activity of the underlying cortical areas of the brain and to have remarkable results even in long-standing disabilities of various kinds.

RYODORAKU

There is a long tradition of acupuncture in Japan. Ryodoraku is a Japanese electrical method, which depends on the Neuro-meter mentioned on page 118. The technique depends on measuring the electrical resistance at 12 points in the wrists and ankles and comparing the values found with those considered to be normal. On the basis of these readings a diagnosis and acupuncture prescription are arrived at and treatment is given using the same machine, which emits a current as well as measuring resistance.

REFERENCES

Brown, M. L., Ulett, G. A. and Stern, J. A. (1974). Acupuncture loci: techniques for location. *American Journal of Chinese Medicine*, **2**, 64–74.

Kenyon, J. N. (1983a). *Modern Techniques of Acupuncture*, p. 65 *et seq*. Thorsons Publications, Wellingborough.

ibid. (1983b). p. 82 *et seq*.

Needham, J. and Gwei-Djen, L. (1980). *Celestial Lancets: A History and Rationale of Acupuncture and Moxa*, pp. 187–8. Cambridge University Press, Cambridge.

Oleson, T. L., Kroening, R. J. and Bresler, D. E. (1980). An experimental evaluation of auricular diagnosis: the somatotopic mapping of musculoskeletal pain at ear acupuncture points. *Pain*, **8**, 217–29.

Reichmanis, M. A. A. and Becker, R. D. (1976). DC skin conductance variation at acupuncture loci. *American Journal of Chinese Medicine*, **4**, 69–72.

Wall, P. and Melzack, R. (1984). *A Textbook of Pain*, p. 697. Churchill Livingstone, Edinburgh.

Chapter Nine

TRANSCUTANEOUS ELECTRICAL NERVE STIMULATION

Transcutaneous electrical nerve stimulation (TENS) is in many ways similar to acupuncture and probably works by similar methods. Like acupuncture, it has a long history – the Romans, it seems, recommended touching an electric torpedo fish as a treatment for rheumatism – but the modern version goes back to the 1960s. The basic idea is to apply a small electric current to nerves through the skin; it is possible to stimulate any nerve in this way down to a depth of about 4cm. The nerves used may be the large nerves in the arm or leg or any of the superficial skin nerves. The apparatus consists of a small battery-powered stimulator putting out a continuous train of electrical impulses, which are applied to the patient's skin through silicone rubber pads (Fig. 9/1). Contact is ensured by the use of electrode jelly or karaya gum (which also sticks the electrode to the skin). The patient adjusts the intensity of stimulation to a level at which a not unpleasant tingling sensation is felt in the area supplied by the nerve or nerves in question. If the treatment is successful, she will experience partial or complete relief of pain while the machine is switched on, and this relief may continue for some hours after the end of treatment. In the best cases TENS may produce a complete cure, but as a rule it has to be continued at intervals indefinitely.

As with other treatment there is a considerable placebo response to TENS. However, the initial true response rate in

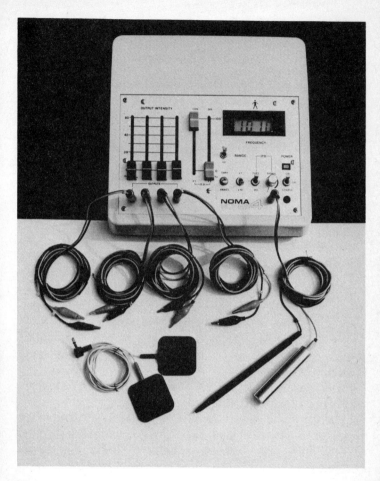

Fig. 9/1 The NOMA Super 4 transcutaneous electrical nerve stimulation machine (*courtesy* P. H. Medical, Weybridge)

suitable kinds of pain is about 60 or 70 per cent – about the same as for acupuncture – and though there is a tendency for the response rate to fall with time, about 30 per cent of patients will continue to get good relief indefinitely.

Among the kinds of pain that may respond to TENS are low

back pain, osteoarthritis, post-herpetic neuralgia, peripheral nerve injury, phantom limb pain, stump pain and some cases of unexplained abdominal pain. It is usually the treatment to try first in pain due to nerve injury; for example, causalgia and stump pain. TENS is of little use in central (thalamic) pain, peripheral neuropathy and psychogenic pain.

These are all examples of chronic pain states, but TENS can also be useful in acute pain; for example, acute lumbago. It has been used after surgery, the electrodes being placed around the incision; here it often reduces the patient's discomfort and her need for postoperative narcotic drugs. TENS is widely used in Sweden during the early stages of labour. It has been applied very successfully to relieve the pain of fractured ribs, and for toothache: dentists have used it as an analgesic in acute pulpitis.

Although normally thought of as a treatment for pain, TENS can logically be tried in any situation where stimulation of nerves is thought to be useful. For example, I have used it successfully to treat a patient suffering from clonic facial spasm (see p. 102) and it can also be used to relax limb spasticity due, for example, to multiple sclerosis. Professor Kaada's use of TENS to treat leg ulcers and other circulatory disorders, discussed below, is yet another application to non-painful disorders (Kaada, 1986).

From what I have said it will be evident that TENS is in many ways similar to acupuncture and should be thought of whenever acupuncture produces an improvement that is only temporary. However, acupuncture and TENS are not precisely equivalent to each other; some patients respond to TENS who do not respond to acupuncture and vice versa. The advantages of TENS are that it is painless, so can be used on patients who are afraid of acupuncture, and it can be applied at home by the patient herself. The disadvantages are chiefly the expense and, usually, the need to continue treatment indefinitely. TENS is very safe, but it should be avoided in patients who have a demand pacemaker implanted, since these pacemakers work by detecting the electrical impulses from the patient's heart, which they use as a signal to stimulate the heart, and it is possible that they might mistake impulses from the TENS machine for cardiac activity. Theoretically, there is a risk of causing cardiac arrhythmias by stimulating the vagus nerve or by passing current across the chest, and spasm of the vocal cords might be caused by stimulating the recurrent laryngeal nerves. No such cases have been reported, but it seems safest to avoid passing the current across the chest (for example, from one arm to the other) and not to stimulate the region of the carotid sinus.

A few patients become allergic to the rubber of which the electrodes are made; electrodes of different materials are available or one can make one's own out of aluminium foil. A more common reason for skin irritation to develop under the electrodes, however, is using insufficient electrode jelly, which leads to poor contact and excessive electrical transmission at just a few points.

The mechanism by which TENS works is not fully understood, but Melzack and Wall (1984) believe that it depends on mechanisms situated mainly in the brainstem. There are nerve cells here (the reticular formation) that receive input from many parts of the body and, in turn, 'project' to many parts of the spinal cord and brain. Moreover, if points within the reticular formation are stimulated electrically, analgesia can result in different areas of the body. Possibly these points can be activated by electrical stimulation of particular body areas.

PRACTICAL ASPECTS OF TENS

Placement of electrodes

The siting of the electrodes is very important in TENS. There are several possibilities.

1. The simplest method is merely to place one on each side of the painful area. This is what is usually done in post-herpetic neuralgia, for example.
2. Another method is to place the electrodes over a major nerve supplying the painful area. Thus, in sciatica they could be placed over the sciatic nerve itself, or on two sides of the leg.
3. The electrodes may be placed over the painful dermatome.

4. TPs, if present, may be used.
5. The electrodes may be placed over the spine, several segments above the painful dermatome or myotome.

It is necessary to spend some time experimenting with different electrode placements if the first one tried does not give good results, since positioning the electrodes may be crucial for success.

Apparatus

The various machines used for TENS emit electrical pulses of different kinds. A biphasic wave has theoretical advantages but is more difficult to generate, so most machines use a rectangular waveform in which there is a square-wave positive component followed by a brief negative component. The *amplitude* of the pulse wave is adjustable on all the machines, and is set by the patient to give a comfortable tingling feeling.

The *duration* of the pulse (pulse width) is another variable which can be adjusted on some machines; however, on most it is set by the manufacturer, usually to about 0.2–0.4 milliseconds (200–400 microseconds). If the duration is longer than about 1 millisecond the patient will feel an unpleasant burning sensation.

The third variable, which is always adjustable, is the frequency of the pulses; this used to be given in cycles per second but is now called hertz (Hz). Thus a machine set at 80Hz puts out 80 pulses per second.

The total amount of electricity emitted by a TENS machine depends on all three variables together; increasing the pulse duration, for example, while leaving the other variables the same, will increase the total amount of electricity received by the patient and thus the strength of the stimulation. (It will also shorten the life of the battery.)

The frequency at which TENS is used is very important. There are two main modes: slow stimulation at 2–6Hz (sometimes referred to as acupuncture-like stimulation because this is approximately the frequency of manual stimulation of needles) and fast stimulation, usually in the range 60–140Hz. Although a few reports have favoured the use of slow stimulation, most have found fast stimulation to be better. There may be quite a narrow frequency 'window' in which the treatment will work for any given patient, so as with electrode replacement it is important to experiment. The best frequency is usually in the range 40–80Hz. Most of the TENS machines on the market in the UK at present do not permit exact setting of the frequency; the control knob usually has arbitrary numbers so the frequency has to be estimated aproximately from the known range of the machine.

Slow stimulation, if used, should be strong enough to produce a muscle twitch. (Fast stimulation does not produce a twitch because it is above the rate to which the muscles can respond.) Slow stimulation of this kind can be uncomfortable, and it is better to use a machine which puts out 'bursts' of brief pulses at, say, two bursts per second.

An interesting application of slow stimulation has recently been described by Professor B. Kaada (1986). His method is to place the electrodes over LI 4 and SI 3 on one hand and to stimulate so as to cause a muscle contraction at a rate of 2Hz for 30–45 minutes, 2 or 3 times daily. A 'burst' machine is usually used. Kaada finds that this technique produces widespread increases in skin temperature, which come on after 15–30 minutes and last for 2–6 hours. He has used his treatment successfully in patients suffering from chronic leg ulcers or pressure sores which had failed to heal, sometimes for years, and also in patients with circulation problems caused by diabetes, venous insufficiency, arteriosclerosis, thromboangiitis obliterans and Raynaud's disease. He suggests that these effects may be due to changes in the nervous control of the blood vessels in the skin or to release of chemical substances that cause vasodilatation.

Dr L. M. Rapson, of Toronto, has used slow TENS as a substitute for acupuncture. She applies the current through cottonwool buds soaked in saline to render them conductive; brief (5–10 seconds) stimulation is used at 4Hz. The brevity of the treatment is remarkable but Dr Rapson believes that the nervous system adapts very rapidly to stimulation and that all the effects of acupuncture are produced within the first few seconds. This treatment is pain free and, like ordinary TENS, can be applied by the patient at home (Rapson, 1986).

USING TENS

Probably the commonest reason for the failure of TENS to work is that the patient is not using it properly. It is therefore essential for the doctor or physiotherapist to spend a good deal of time explaining the method to the patient and making sure that she understands how to use it. Whenever possible I like to admit patients to hospital for a week or so to get them started; this also allows me to try different settings and electrode positions and to assess the patient's response for myself. Initially the machine is left on all day and sometimes all night as well; later this can usually be reduced to a few hours each day. If the treatment seems to be working I then send the patient out to try the machine at home for a month or so; this is important in order to detect the placebo responders, who will cease to obtain benefit after about six weeks. Provided the response is maintained the patient is then asked to buy a machine for herself. (There is no regular National Health Service mechanism for supplying these machines.)

The machines vary in price, but at present (1986) £60 is about the norm. There are a number of satisfactory machines on the market; the MicroTENS is a good example (Fig. 9/2). It is well made and robust, and is small, light and easy to carry about, so that patients can continue with their normal activities during stimulation. The frequency range is from 15–120Hz; a model with 'burst' facility is available but the pulse width is not adjustable. The principal disadvantage of the MicroTENS is that the knobs controlling amplitude and frequency are close together and look exactly alike, so are liable to be confused by elderly patients. As with most TENS machines, the controls are small and fiddly and difficult to manipulate with arthritic fingers.

Another good machine is the Staodyn. This comes from America and is twice the price of most British machines, but it does allow adjustment of the pulse width. There is a version

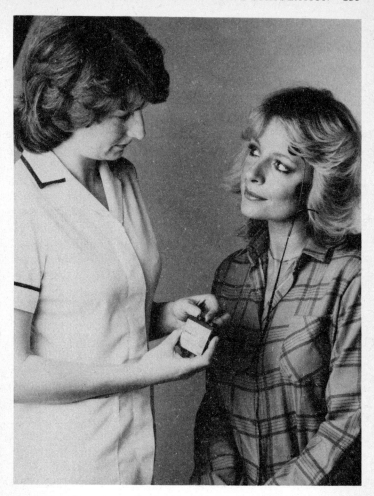

Fig. 9/2 The MicroTENS transcutaneous electrical nerve stimulation machine (*courtesy* P. H. Medical, Weybridge)

that has a 4-channel output. I have found that some patients seem to respond better to the Staodyn than to other machines, perhaps because of the precise characteristics of its electrical output, but for most patients a less expensive machine will be just as satisfactory.

CLINICAL USES

TENS is worth trying for any patient who responds to acupuncture but only for short periods. In addition, there are certain problems, such as post-herpetic neuralgia, which do not respond well to acupuncture but quite often do respond to TENS.

A particularly interesting application of TENS is to unexplained abdominal pain. Some patients suffer chronic abdominal pain, either spontaneously or following an operation, but in spite of the most extensive investigations no cause for the pain is found. When the pain follows surgery it is often attributed to 'adhesions', but it is very doubtful that these are really the cause. Whenever abdominal surgery is carried out adhesions – that is, fibrous connections – form between the peritoneum covering the abdominal organs as a normal part of the healing process, but except in the rare cases in which they compress and obstruct the bowel there is no reason to think that they give rise to pain.

It seems more likely, in fact, that abdominal pain of this kind is in many cases yet another example of a 'pain pattern' becoming established in the nervous system. This explains why it quite often responds to TENS. The electrodes are placed on two sides of the painful area and stimulation is continued for several hours.

TENS can be thought of as a logical extension of acupuncture. It probably works by much the same mechanisms and it can be used to treat much the same kinds of problem, though there are some differences. I think it likely that the next few years will see some exciting new developments in TENS. One pointer to this is Professor Kaada's work on vascular disorders. Another is the development, in Canada and elsewhere, of new types of stimulator designed to make use of our increasing knowledge of the ways the nervous system functions. This is just one more example of how the ancient practice of acupuncture is being taken up and given new applications today.

REFERENCES

Kaada, B. (1986). Treatment of peripheral ischaemia and chronic ulceration by transcutaneous nerve stimulation (TNS). *Acupuncture in Medicine*, **3**, 30.

Melzack, R. and Wall, P. (1984). Acupuncture and transcutaneous nerve stimulation. *Postgraduate Medical Journal*, **60**, 893–6.

Rapson, L. M. (1986). Transcutaneous electrical stimulation in pain treatment: some innovative approaches. (Paper presented at the Second World Congress of Scientific Acupuncture, London.)

Chapter Ten
CLINICAL RESEARCH IN ACUPUNCTURE

A considerable amount of research in acupuncture has appeared, some of it of rather dubious quality. I do not intend to review it all here, but the Bibliography will give some indications for further reading. However, I think it is worth while to outline briefly what I think are the main problems confronting researchers in acupuncture and which are largely peculiar to acupuncture.

Most of these problems centre on what kind of controls to use. To the mildly interested onlooker with no particular knowledge of acupuncture this seems fairly simple; surely all that needs to be done is to compare 'real' acupuncture with random needling at non-acupuncture points. If a difference between the two treatments is demonstrated, fine; acupuncture works. If not, it is 'just a placebo'.

Unfortunately, things are not so simple. Owing to the phenomenon of diffuse noxious inhibitory control, there will be some therapeutic response from random needling, over and above the placebo effect. So-called placebo acupuncture, therefore, is not a true placebo at all but another form of treatment.

There is another difficulty attached to the idea of placebo acupuncture. Suppose 20 patients are treated with 'real' acupuncture by Dr A., an experienced acupuncturist, and another 20 with 'placebo' acupuncture by Dr B., who knows nothing about acupuncture. We cannot validly compare the outcomes, because we cannot assume that the two doctors possess equally potent personalities in terms of their placebo effects. But if, to get round this difficulty, we allow Dr A. to treat both groups, a different problem arises. Dr A. cannot be neutral about what he is doing; whether he wishes to or not, he will probably communicate something of his own beliefs and prejudices to his patients (at least, we cannot assume that he will not). Dr B., on the other hand, may not produce the same therapeutic response as Dr A., and his treatment would not be regarded as valid acupuncture by most medical acupuncturists.

Even if, for the sake of argument, we grant that Dr A. can maintain a completely impassive attitude that gives nothing away, we still are not out of the wood. Difficulties now arise concerning the acupuncture itself. How far away from the 'correct' site are the placebo needles to be placed? How deeply are they to be inserted? How much stimulation is to be given, and is teh chi to be obtained? In short, there is a large range of possible variations in the way acupuncture is performed, and this makes comparison of different types of needling almost impossible.

Probably the nearest one can get to placebo acupuncture is to devise a treatment that the patient will think is needling although in fact it is not. Some years ago in Finland Dr Junnila carried out a study in back pain, in which he put needles into the patients' backs so that they could not see what was happening. Before each insertion he gave the patient's back a quick slap; in the case of the control group he gave the slap but did not insert a needle. In this case the deception was successful but this procedure is obviously not applicable to every trial (personal communication).

Another approach, used by Macdonald (1983) and subsequently by other researchers, is to compare acupuncture with mock TENS (that is, a TENS machine with the power switched off). However, it could be argued that mock TENS is not really comparable with acupuncture in placebo power.

In view of all these difficulties many researchers have come to the conclusion that placebo acupuncture is not a real possibility, and that a better idea is to compare acupuncture with other treatment. In such cases it is very desirable that the results of treatment, at least, are assessed by an independent judge rather than by the acupuncturist himself. This was the procedure adopted by Dr Loh and his colleagues in their headache study (Loh et al, 1984).

Another solution, which was adopted by Dr Junnila (1986), is to dispense with any kind of control group and instead to follow up a group of treated patients for a long time; that is, to use the patients as their own controls. This is a valid way of doing research provided the follow-up methods are adequate and it can yield valuable information that is not afforded by other kinds of study.

Although there is now quite a large body of research literature on acupuncture, it is variable in quality and much of it has been published in rather obscure journals that are probably inaccessible to many would-be readers. Fortunately, however, two fairly comprehensive articles have appeared in recent years in *Pain*. Lewith and Machin (1983) reviewed 32 papers and concluded that the response rate is about 30 per cent for placebo, 50 per cent for sham acupuncture, and 70 per cent for real acupuncture. Most of the published trials, they believe, would not be capable of detecting differences of this order, hence one cannot necessarily conclude from these trials that acupuncture is merely a placebo. They suggest that instead of comparing acupuncture and placebo it would be better to analyse the time for which a patient obtains relief from a given treatment.

More recently, Vincent and Richardson (1986) reviewed 40 studies. They, too, found serious shortcomings in most of the reports, but they concluded that there is good evidence for the short-term effectiveness of acupuncture in relieving a number of types of pain (mainly headache and back pain but also a number of other painful disorders). They found the short-term success rate to be 50–80 per cent – higher, that is, than the expected placebo response rate of 30–35 per cent. The good initial response was not so well maintained, however, unless patients received booster treatments at intervals; this of course accords with what is found in ordinary clinical practice. No conclusions could be drawn about whether certain points are more effective than others.

Like Lewith and Machin, Vincent and Richardson are sceptical about the value of double-blind trials for assessing the efficacy of acupuncture. They argue that single-blind trials in which the outcome is assessed by an independent judge are adequate 'provided efforts are made to monitor independently the impact of non-specific effects and/or ensure that they do not vary between groups'. They also make a plea, which I would certainly endorse, for authors of research papers to give as much information as possible about what they actually did (number of sessions, duration and frequency of stimulation, whether teh chi was sought, method of point selection, and so forth).

In spite of the difficulties that attend the carrying out of good research in acupuncture, it is very important that it be done. Acupuncture has come and gone a number of times in the West, and there is no guarantee that it will not fall into disuse yet again. That would be a pity, for it has a valuable, if limited, contribution to make to medicine. At present it is at least part-way across the gulf that separates charlatanry from science in the minds of doctors, but if it is to complete the transition it will have to produce evidence that it works.

By itself, however, that will not be enough. It will also be necessary to produce some kind of rational account of *how* it might work. This will have to be a physiological explanation. In the case of pain a basis for explaining at least the short-term effects of acupuncture exists, but it is more difficult to account for the long-term effects and still more difficult to find a framework to accommodate the role of acupuncture as a treatment for non-painful disorders. However, I do not believe that it is impossible to do so.

REFERENCES

Junnila, S.Y.T. (1986). Acupuncture for long time treatment of headache in National Health Centres. (Paper presented at the Second World Congress of Scientific Acupuncture, London.)

Lewith, G. T. and Machin, D. (1983). On the evaluation of the clinical effects of acupuncture. *Pain*, **16**, 111–27.

Loh, L. et al (1984). Acupuncture versus medical treatment for migraine and muscle tension headaches. *Journal of Neurology, Neurosurgery and Psychiatry*, **17**, 333–7.

Macdonald, A. J. R. et al (1983). Superficial acupuncture in the relief of chronic low back pain. *Annals of the Royal College of Surgeons of England*, **65**, 44–6.

Vincent, C. A. and Richardson, P. H. (1986). The evaluation of therapeutic acupuncture: concepts and methods. *Pain*, **24**, 1–13; 15–40.

BIBLIOGRAPHY

TRADITIONAL CHINESE MEDICINE

Anon (1973). *An Outline of Chinese Acupuncture*. The Academy of Traditional Chinese Medicine, Peking.

A textbook of acupuncture as practised today in China. The book is practical and is evidently intended for practitioners with little or no previous medical training (barefoot doctors). Recommended as a description of modern Chinese acupuncture 'straight from the horse's mouth'.

Kaptchuk, T. J. (1983). *Chinese Medicine: The Web Has No Weaver*. (Rider) Hutchinson Publishing Group Ltd, London.

A good readable account of Chinese medicine (mainly acupuncture) by an American who spent a number of years in China. Though an enthusiast for the Chinese system, Kaptchuk maintains a sense of proportion and his book, though detailed, is clear and readable. Probably the best introduction to traditional Chinese medicine at present available in English.

Macdonald, A. (1984). *Acupuncture: From Ancient Art to Modern Medicine*, George Allen and Unwin, London.

A description of mainly traditional acupuncture from the point of view of a Western doctor who practises scientific acupuncture. The traditional ideas are assessed in the light of modern knowledge. The book is intended for the non-medical reader.

Needham, J. and Gwei-Djen, L. (1980). *Celestial Lancets: A History and Rationale of Acupuncture and Moxa*. Cambridge University Press, Cambridge.

The fullest and most scholarly account of traditional acupuncture available. It also contains a great deal of information about modern scientific work on acupuncture. It is essential reading for anyone who wishes to study the subject in depth.

Newnham, R. (1971). *About Chinese*. Penguin Books, Harmondsworth.

A short, very readable, introduction to the Chinese language for the non-learner. It sheds light on the difficulties faced by the translator and helps the Western reader to appreciate the conceptual gulf that separates Chinese and Occidental thought.

Needham, J. (ed. Ronan, C. A.) (1980). *The Shorter Science and Civilisation in China*, vol. 1. Cambridge University Press, Cambridge.

This is an abridgement of the first two volumes of Joseph Needham's monumental work. It presents, in a readily accessible form, a fascinating wealth of material on the background to traditional Chinese medicine.

SCIENTIFIC ACUPUNCTURE

Cyriax, J. (1982). *Textbook of Orthopaedic Medicine*, 8th edition, Baillière Tindall, London.

Cyriax did not believe in acupuncture and he insisted uncompromisingly on the view that there must always be an anatomical lesion in musculoskeletal pain; nevertheless his book is useful to the medical acupuncturist for its discussion of techniques of examination.

Grieve, G. P. (1981). *Common Vertebral Joint Problems*. Churchill Livingstone, Edinburgh.

An exhaustive review of its subject, with nearly 1400 references. Grieve is a physiotherapist and his main therapeutic interest is in manipulation. He does discuss acupuncture briefly, but the main value of his book for the medical acupuncturist is its discussion of applied anatomy and various kinds of clinical presentation of back disorders.

Mann, F. (1980). *The Treatment of Disease by Acupuncture*, 3rd edition. Heinemann Books, London.

Melzack, R. and Wall, P. D. (1982). *The Challenge of Pain*. Penguin Books, Harmondsworth.

An exposition of these authors' very influential theory of pain, apparently written for the non-medical reader but containing a certain amount of technical material. Essential reading for anyone wishing to understand the modern scientific approach to acupuncture.

Travell, J. G. and Simons, D. G. (1983). *Myofascial Pain and Dysfunction: The Trigger Point Manual*. Williams and Wilkins, Baltimore/London.

The essential source book for the trigger point concept. It is required reading for anyone intending to practise scientific acupuncture. This is the first of two planned volumes and deals with the upper half of the body. The second volume is promised but has not yet appeared.

Wall, P. D. and Melzack, R. (jt. eds.) (1984). *A Textbook of Pain*. Churchill Livingstone, Edinburgh.

A comprehensive survey of modern ideas about the causation and treatment of pain. There are chapters on TENS and acupuncture.

INDEX